NO MORE LOSS

Preventing Suicide by Building a Healthy Body, Mind, and Spirit

*Sue —
You were beautifully created by our Lord —
Never forget that!
Mary Rose*

NO MORE LOSS

Preventing Suicide by Building a Healthy Body, Mind, and Spirit

By Nancy L. Rose, NTP, CSCS, CHFS, CGP

This book is not intended as a substitute for the medical advice of a physician(s). The reader should regularly consult a physician in matters relating to his/her health and particularly with respect to any symptoms that may require diagnosis or medical attention. The author and publisher specifically disclaim any liability, loss, or risk, personal, or otherwise, that is incurred as a consequence, directly or indirectly of the use and application of any of the contents of this book.

Copyright © 2015 by Nancy L. Rose

All rights reserved. This book or any portion thereof may not be reproduced or used in any manner whatsoever without the express written permission of the author except for the use of brief quotations in a book review or scholarly journal.

First Printing: 2015

ISBN-10: 163318496X
ISBN-13: 9781633184961

Get At The Roots Weight Loss, LLC.
388 East Main St.
Branford, CT 06405

www.GetAtTheRoots.com

Ordering Information:

Special discounts are available on quantity purchases by corporations, associations, educators, and others. For details, contact the publisher at info@getattheroots.com.

Cover Photo by s.j.bridgeman photography (www.sarahbridgemanphoto.com)
Cover Design by Tru Blu Grafix (www.trublugrafix.com)
Editing by Kimberly Huther (www.wordsmithproofreading.com)

Author's Note

I've known for quite some time now that I wanted to share my story with the world, in hopes of helping others find freedom from mental illness, as I have. I began writing my story years ago, but was stirred in my spirit to finally begin the process to bring my story to others when I heard the news of Matthew Warren taking his life in April of 2013. Matthew was the son of Pastor Rick and Kay Warren of Saddleback Church, who have several churches in California. Rick Warren wrote the book, *The Purpose Driven Life*, along with many other books as well. Rick's book touched my heart when I read it years ago, and really made me think about my purpose in life. Many times we go through things that are leading us to what we were placed on this earth to do. My life experiences have brought me to my life purpose. I know with all my heart that my purpose is to help educate others in the areas of health (nutrition, fitness, spiritual, and emotional) in order to help others to get their bodies and minds healthy. My true desire is to help others find freedom from the torment of mental illness. After this terrible news, I was certain it was time to get my message out there, and so I began to write.

In August of 2014, Robin Williams took his life. What I knew to be true of my purpose was further driven into my soul as I heard the sad news. I must get my message out there. If it helps to save even one life, it is worth it to me. I hope and pray with all my heart that multitudes of people are helped with the information in this book as I have been.

This book is dedicated to

Matthew Warren

Robin Williams

And to all who have lost their lives to suicide

May we get to a place of No More Loss.
May those in need be helped and find joy and freedom from mental illness. May God bless those who have lost loved ones to suicide and bring healing to your life.

Table of Contents

Acknowledgement ix
Book Overview x
Introduction 1
Chapter 1: My Story 7
Chapter 2: Building Optimal Mental Health 23
Chapter 3: Spiritual Health 25
Chapter 4: Emotional Health 34
Chapter 5: A Healthy Nervous System 42
Chapter 6: Building a Healthy Mind Nutritionally 51
Chapter 7: Optimal Mental Health Nutrition Plan 61
Chapter 8: Breakdown of Food Choices & Meals 79
Chapter 9: Digestive Health 100
Chapter 10: Hydration 111
Chapter 11: Microbiome & Sleep 114
Chapter 12: Liver Health 125
Chapter 13: Hormone Health 132
Chapter 14: Detoxification 149
Chapter 15: Specific Nutrients 158
Chapter 16: Physical Fitness 166
Chapter 17: Other Therapies 172
References 175
Quick Reference Shopping List 186

Nancy Rose

Acknowledgements

First and foremost, I am thankful to my Lord and Savior, Jesus Christ, for leading me to freedom from mental torment and giving me the wisdom to write this book.

I am thankful to my family and friends who have offered tremendous support in completing this project. I am especially thankful to my siblings, Bette Pilecki and Loretta Miller for reviewing and offering valuable feedback. I am also very thankful for my life coach, Peggy Hoime, who has been instrumental in encouraging me and offering me valuable wisdom during this time of my life. I am thankful to my friend, Ginny Brestelli, for her valuable feedback and continuous prayer support. Many people have prayed for the completion of this book and I appreciate every one of you! For all of you, I am truly grateful.

To my Aunt Suzie Snelgrove and prayer warrior siblings, Loretta Miller, James Rose, and Bette Pilecki, I am forever grateful for you and blessed that God gave you to me as my family and friends for life! Your prayers have changed the course of my life and helped me through so many difficult times.

To my amazing son, Jonathan, who has been one of the main motivators in my life to gain freedom from mental illness. You are truly a gift from God to me.

Book Overview

This book addresses five components of healing in order to optimize mental health.

Spiritual Healing

Your life is valuable! You were created for a purpose! You have worth! When you discover the purpose that God placed you on this earth for everything changes; your whole outlook on life changes.

Emotional Healing

If you have experienced trauma in your life you are not alone. You will learn six keys to unlocking emotional trauma to help bring healing to your life.

Neurological Healing

The brain sends messages to the rest of the body via the nervous system. If nerves are not able to properly relay messages, there can problems anywhere in the body including the brain. A healthy nervous system is vital for optimal mental and physical health.

Nutritional Healing

Did you know that the health of your gut could be directly affecting your brain? Did you know that your moods can be greatly impacted by your blood sugar levels? That being exposed to toxins can lead to mental health problems? That food allergies can create sadness, hyperactivity, or anxiety? You will learn about all of this and more…

Physical Fitness

Exercising at the appropriate intensity is good for the body and brain and causes the release of your feel good hormones, your endorphins. You will learn how over-exercising can be hindering your state of mind. I will also help you to discover the perfect exercise for you, to bring life to your body and health to your brain.

Introduction

Let me start by saying that the methods for treating mental illness in this country are less than ideal. Although the methods have changed drastically over the years, the truth is that the treatment for the mentally ill is still not wonderful and potentially dangerous. According to the documentary, Psychiatry: An Industry of Death, ***"there have been twice as many people who have been killed in psychiatric hospitals than all the wars combined since 1776."***[1] The treatment of the mentally ill has been utterly disturbing. If you are unaware of how the mentally ill have been treated in the past, and how they are treated today, read the book, *Mad in America* by Robert Whitaker. Trust me when I tell you that, after reading that book, you will be sick to your stomach with the methods that have been used to treat the mentally ill. Although things have changed from torture to drugging, the methods are still not ideal by any stretch of the imagination. The use of psychotropic medication to treat mental illness fails in one very important area: Getting At The Root of the Problem. This book is intended to help bring out root issues that will hinder your ability to live with a normal functioning brain. If you want to get at the root of your mental health problems once and for all, please read through this entire book. I pray that as you do, God would lead you to the answers you need to find freedom from mental anguish, and bring life and health to your body and brain.

Suicide Statistics

The most current data I could find regarding suicide statistics comes from the year 2012. In 2012, an average of one person every 13 minutes committed suicide in the United States, which was the 10th ranking cause of death in the U.S. overall, but the 2nd leading cause of death for the young. Thirteen million adults attempted suicide, which equates to one attempt every 31 seconds.[2]

Ninety percent of those who attempt suicide have a diagnosed mental illness, most common of which are depression, bipolar disorder, schizophrenia, personality disorder, anxiety disorders, and eating disorders.[3] It is clear that suicide is a major concern that needs to be addressed. Too many are losing their loved ones to suicide. Many are feeling hopeless and that there is no real solution or effective treatment to prevent this. Ask anyone who has lost a loved one to suicide if they would go back and do anything that they could to prevent it and they would. The problem isn't that there is no prevention. The problem is that the standard means of prevention is medication and psychotherapy. This clearly is not working well. Remember that 90% of those who commit suicide have been diagnosed with a mental illness.[3] This tells me that most have sought help at one point or another but, ultimately, that help failed them. Many are not aware of other methods of preventing mental health problems. Most are unaware of the many things that contribute to the deterioration of mental health. My goal is to bring awareness to some of the underlying causes of mental illness and help lead you in a direction to help heal and restore optimal brain function.

Medication Isn't Working

In the major psychiatric conditions of bipolar disorder and schizophrenia, it is often deemed that individuals need to be medicated for the rest of their life. There is no cure. They are often put on a cocktail of medications that frequently stop working and need to be constantly adjusted. My hope is to change your opinion of these very things. I believe that an individual can heal from this, that there are root issues and, once these issues are corrected, an individual can live a life free from mental illness. I want to pose the idea that there is a cure!

Through the years, as I studied on these topics, I met many people who had been diagnosed with mental illness (major depression, bipolar disorder, and schizophrenia). All of these individuals were on one or multiple psychotropic medications. I would often ask them how they felt the medication was working for them. I got a varied response. Some believed the medication was working, others thought it was helping a little, and still others did not feel it was really working. I would then continue to ask them how they felt. I would ask them if they were still experiencing symptoms and almost always it was, "Yes!" Mental illness is diagnosed based on a list of symptoms as spelled out in the Diagnostic and Statistical Manual of Mental Disorders (DSMV).[4] If you fit the description, you are then diagnosed and often prescribed medication. The problem that I saw was that this medication did not seem to really be helping these individuals, at least not enough, in my opinion, to make their quality of life better than without it. I did have a few individuals swear by their anti-depressant, but often really wondered if any of these medicines were truly helping. Psychologist Dr. Irving Kirsch had that same question, and wrote an entire book about it titled, *The Emperor's New Drugs: Exploding the Antidepressant Myth*, after he teamed with a grad student, Guy Sapirstein, to do a meta-analysis of all the research on anti-depressants. The meta-analysis was done only on anti-depressants and not on other psychotropic medications. The conclusion that he comes to in the book is very telling, in my opinion.

"Although many depressed patients improve when given medication, so do many who are given a placebo, and the difference between the drug response and the placebo response is not all that great. What the published studies really indicate is that most of the improvement shown by depressed people when they take anti-depressants is due to the placebo effect." [5]

The results from the meta-analysis showed that anti-depressants helped to a degree, but the placebo also helped almost as much. Psychotherapy had the greatest benefit (slightly more than medication), and doing nothing did not help much at all.[5] You could conclude that the effect of the anti-depressant is a placebo effect. Others certainly may view this differently, but I agree with Dr. Kirsch's conclusion.

I believe that this shows that simply the hope of being helped, whether it is from medication, placebo, or therapy has a profound impact on how well someone will do. The power of the mind is amazing. The key is in continuing to provide hope through many avenues of healing. In this book you will learn about the many different areas to address in order to optimize your success in obtaining a healthy mind. As with everything, it starts in the power of your thoughts. Our thoughts impact our brain chemistry, hormones, and a cascade of processes in the body that can benefit us or cause harm.

Medication Is Risky

While writing this book, I had the television on in the background, and was interrupted when I heard a commercial. I had heard multiple commercials of similar origin to this in the past, but this time I decided to listen more intently. This was a commercial for a medication promoted for bipolar depression. Like most commercials for prescription medications, this had a list of potential side-effects of the medication. I cannot figure out how anyone would truly want to even risk taking these medications after hearing this, but obviously many individuals are. Here are just some potential side-effects associated with the use of psychotropic medication, taken from the National Institute of Mental Health:

Anti-psychotics: drowsiness, dizziness, blurred vision, rapid heartbeat, sensitivity to sun, skin rashes, menstrual problems for women, weight gain, rigidity, persistent muscle spasms, tremors, restlessness, tardive dyskinesia.[6]

Anti-depressants: headaches, nausea, drowsiness, agitation, sexual problems, dry mouth, constipation, bladder problems, blurred vision.[6]

Lithium (used as a mood stabilizer for bipolar disorder): loss of coordination, excessive thirst, frequent urination, blackouts, seizures, slurred speech, fast, slow, irregular or pounding heartbeat, hallucinations, changes in vision, itching, swelling.[6]

Medications for ADHD: acting more subdued or withdrawn, feeling helpless, hopeless or worthless, new or worsening depression, thinking or talking about hurting oneself, extreme worry, agitation, panic attacks, trouble sleeping, irritability, aggressive or violent behavior, acting without thinking, extreme increase in activity or talking, frenzied/abnormal excitement, any sudden or unusual changes in behavior.[6]

The use of anti-depressant medication can also potentially increase the risk of suicide and to me is something not worth the risk. Unfortunately, I believe many people are unaware of the potential dangers of psychotropic medications. Sometimes these side-effects are not even discussed when being prescribed. Many people believe that medication is their only source of hope. I also believe many people are becoming discouraged by not getting true help, are suffering side-effects, and are looking for alternative treatments to conventional medicine. The purpose of this book is to offer hope outside of the standard model for mental health treatment.

Withdrawal From Medication Is Just As Risky

Harvard-trained psychiatrist, Dr. Peter Breggin has spent decades changing the way others view mental health and the use of psychotropic medication. He has written several books on the topic including: *Talking Back to Prozac* (1994), *Medication Madness: The Role of Psychiatric Drugs in Cases of Violence, Suicide, and Crime* (2008), and *Psychiatric Drug Withdrawal: A Guide for Prescribers, Therapists, Patients, and Their Families* (2013). Dr. Breggins is a medical expert in cases involving malpractice and the adverse side-effects of psychotropic medications. I highly recommend reading some of his books to understand both the dangers of taking psychotropic drugs as well as the dangers of withdrawing from them.

If you are currently on psychotropic medication, it is very important that you seek professional help if you are looking to get off of your medication, as withdrawal can cause devastating and life-threatening problems. I cannot emphasize enough the importance of working with a professional trained in withdrawing from psychotropic medication. If you are on any psychotropic medication, please **do not attempt to withdraw without the help of an experienced clinician.**

There Is Hope

It seems as though we are hearing more and more about suicides, and it saddens me, as there is so much we can do to prevent it. Unfortunately it is not as simple a fix as the world has tried to make it with medication and psychotherapy. We have proven that this is NOT working. Our bodies are so intricate that it takes so much more, but is still completely doable and possible. It won't happen overnight but, if you take it one day at a time and work on the areas written in this book, there is definite HOPE for a brighter future. A future full of life and joy! Here's to wishing you all that and more!

Chapter 1

My Story

A Crazy Roller Coaster Ride

It's crazy how you view things a whole lot differently when your hormones or brain chemistry are off. When I say crazy – I mean crazy! It's like you are a whole different person who is not able to deal with life or cope. Imagine that. If you have no idea what I am talking about then count yourself blessed – extremely blessed. If you can relate to what I am saying, then you may have experienced moments of craziness, sadness, depression, and/or an inability to cope with life. Maybe those moments lasted for a whole lot longer than a moment and maybe even days, weeks, or months. If you feel this way or someone you love feels this way, you need to read this book.

People think you're crazy, hormonal, or just a depressed or moody person. Maybe you've even believed it. But the truth is, it's not who you are! You were born for greatness! You were born to accomplish many things and to live a joyous, stable, secure, productive, fulfilling life! However, we begin to believe the other is true (we are depressed, moody, hormonal, and crazy) when we are experiencing horrible fluctuations in feelings. What we feel and who we are does not seem to match at times. Why is that? You're told you need medication. You're told you need therapy. You're told you have problems and they need to be talked about. You're told that there is no cure and that you need to live with it; find a way to cope.

I do not agree! There are many things you can and need to do to feel emotionally well. I will first share with you my journey and then lay out the tools of understanding that God led me to, which resulted in my freedom! That sounds good, doesn't it? Wouldn't you like to be free? To feel normal? To feel stable? Secure? To not fear life and to be able to cope? Then read on.....

I was a very timid child, although I never felt stressed. Looking back, I would say that my childhood was GREAT! Fantastic! I could have stayed there my whole life. No worries or cares up until high school at least. I would have liked to stay in 4th grade for the rest of my life. That would have been perfect. Fifth through eighth weren't bad either. I was, however, extremely shy, which seemed to grow worse as I went into high school. I really didn't talk much and didn't have too many friends. To me, I didn't seem to fit in. I was different from the rest. It wasn't cool to me to go to parties. It wasn't cool to swear. I was different. I was a Christian. I'm not saying that no one else was, but I definitely held tight to my faith and beliefs and wasn't interested really in fitting in. I was an athlete, a talented one at that, and that was my in. I made friends through sports, but had very few close friends who I actually shared anything personal with. Again, I was still very quiet. The first time I can remember feeling sadness and overall melancholy was in high school. It wasn't terrible, but I definitely felt the difference. Things grew much worse for me going into college, but no one knew it. I was still shy, and that was certainly noticed. I didn't fit in. If I didn't fit in in high school because I didn't party, I definitely didn't fit in in college. I played Division I volleyball and I just didn't hang out with the team. I had a couple of friends on the team but, again, I was different. I was very repelled by the lifestyle of drinking, hanging out with a bunch of people, promiscuous sex, etc. It was not me, and I'm certainly glad it wasn't. I could have had a lot more problems if it was. Surprisingly, someone with my brain chemistry makeup at the time would most likely have been drawn to it and thank the Lord in heaven that I was not. I believe many people turn to drugs and alcohol to compensate for deficient brain chemistry. Many times it starts with a desire to fit in or to know the unknown, which leads to a deficiency in nutrients and sets the stage for depleted brain chemistry. You will learn how we are all at different stages, based on our health that we inherited from our parents, and so the results are not the same for everyone if they begin drinking. Some who have depleted brain chemistry before they ever drink will suffer the consequences much quicker than others will. This, too, will be explained. But back to my story…for me, drinking was never a problem. I didn't want to drink. I hated it. Apart from a few occasions, which I will share later, I did not drink alcohol.

So what was so bad? Nothing really, observing from the outside in. Looking at my life, you would have thought I had no right to be depressed, sad, or anxious. Life for me was what most people would have thought to be great! I did well in school – received mostly A's. I made the Scholar Athlete Award most years throughout college. I was a talented athlete, playing three sports a year throughout high school, then walking on to a Division I volleyball team as a freshman in college and placing a starting position my first year. I later went on to receive a scholarship to play and, years later, was inducted into my High School Athletic Hall of Fame. I had great parents and siblings. I wasn't abused. My family went to church and my parents were strong Christians when I was young. My father walked away from the church, but my mom remained faithful and was a great prayer warrior. I know I am a product of her prayers and my dad's, too. I married my high school sweetheart right after college. He seemed to be a perfect fit – my family loved him and he seemed to be what I needed. I was a beautiful, athletic girl. My only flaw physically was some acne. That really did bother me a lot, but throughout college volleyball I was the strongest, had the least body fat, and was the quickest on the team. I was not the best player on the team, but I excelled in the strength and conditioning arena, which set the stage for me to get my degree in Exercise Science. I'm not trying to brag here; I want to emphasize that things can be going totally well for someone but they were born with a deficiency or some other factor is in effect to cause an imbalance in neurotransmitters. I simply didn't have a reason to feel the way that I did. Looking at all that, you would say I had no reason to not want to live but, guess what? That is exactly how I felt.

When I was first married, I struggled to find joy, to get the energy to want to do much of anything. Granted, there was some life adjusting to do as I was no longer an athlete on a team. I was still athletic and played basketball in a Lutheran league with my sister. I struggled to find a job that fit with my degree, so that was difficult but we were not struggling financially. In fact, I had been blessed my whole life up to that point to not feel financially deprived in any way. So what was wrong? The answer is in the following pages, but to simplify it - my brain chemistry was off! There were multiple reasons for it, but the simple matter of it all was that my brain was not properly functioning to allow me to feel emotionally well. I don't care how good or bad your life is… without properly functioning brain chemistry, life is not good. Not only is it not good; it's downright torturous. Hence the feelings of wanting to escape it, to end it, to get out of this life!

Honestly, I really didn't know that this was not how all people felt. I didn't know that there was anything wrong with me. I certainly had a hard time coping with things, and I'm not talking about the death of a loved one. I'm talking about coping with getting up in the morning. I'm talking about coping with making a phone call or running errands. It was that bad at times. Unfortunately, I had no idea how to communicate that to others or to my husband. The only thing I could do was react, and most of the time it was silence, crying, or cowering away into my own world. Others may think (probably my husband at the time) that I was just being selfish, that I needed to just snap out of it, to stop being so depressed. I would have thoughts in my head, but I couldn't get them out of my mouth to express how I felt or what was going on within me. I really did not understand it. Something may trigger a feeling and that was it – all the emotions came flooding and no one knew where they came from. Granted, most people never saw this. Most people had no idea. I was quiet. I was beautiful. I felt so insecure. Some others probably thought I was a snob. They may have thought that I knew I was beautiful and couldn't be bothered with them. That was the farthest thing from the truth. I didn't think I was better than anyone. I had no confidence, but you probably wouldn't have picked up on it apart from the shyness.

I felt like I was trapped in my own body and I needed to escape, but I didn't know how. It's a horrible feeling, really. It's this inner turmoil that you can't seem to get rid of. So, here I was a year out of college, newly married, seeking a job and a purpose, but I didn't know that at the time. I found a job in my field at a local fitness center. I was there a very short amount of time and it just didn't fit me well. I wanted to share my knowledge; they wanted me to sell gym memberships. Being the shy person that I was, that really wasn't a good fit. My husband agreed that I should leave that job and look for something else. I looked for a while and kept coming up short. My husband started to get on me about getting a job. So I applied at a place his sister worked at – completely having nothing to do with my field of study. He kept on me so I kept calling and finally they gave me a position. It wasn't pretty. I worked in a "clean" room where I had to go through a process to gown- up to be totally covered and filter media into bottles. Woo hoo! Good use of my degree for sure. Anyhow, I certainly wasn't feeling fulfilled with that job, but at least I had something to do and was making some money. I began on the morning shift and worked four 10-hour days a week. My shift ran from 5 am until 3 pm. That meant I had to get up around 3:30 am to get ready. This was the first mistake of many, and began my sleep deprivation. Sleep is very important to your adrenal glands and to your overall mental health. After a few months, I was switched to the later shift, which ran from 3 pm until 1 am. This, again, was not a good fit for me. Either way, I was messing with my sleep schedule. On top of that, I never saw my husband. This, for me, was a prescription for disaster. Let's recap that I was already struggling with life and then let's add to it sleep deprivation, a low self-esteem, hardly seeing my husband, and what happens? A man at my job starts to show me attention. Here I am with no self-esteem and I can't wear makeup and I have to wear scrubs and this man is attracted to me!?! Out of nowhere, he tells me I'm beautiful and my body chemistry sang a new song. Suddenly my endorphins kicked in and I was feeling on top of the world – suddenly I don't seem to have deficient brain chemistry! I feel great! I want to feel that more. I'm hooked.

It wasn't long before I was doing some crazy things like leaving work in the middle of the shift to take off to Florida with this man and not telling my husband or his wife. Let me just interject that we lived in upstate New York by the Canadian border, so Florida was about a 24-hour drive. We left notes for them; my husband filled out a missing person report; a family member thought I was abducted – certain I would never do something like this and that I must have been forced to write the note; we drive to Florida. Crazy – yes – crazy! What in the heck was I thinking? I was thinking my brain is functioning – maybe not normally – but a whole lot better in this moment and I need more of this. That's exactly what I was thinking. There are physiological changes that occur in the body and brain chemistry due to emotional events, such as the affection of another person, and this can be very powerful. Emotions can go in a positive direction or a negative direction. These definitely felt positive. Give me more, give me more! It felt like these emotions were non-existent at the time or at least hard to come by. Did it mean that I didn't have love for my husband? No, certainly not. What it meant was my brain chemistry was not stable enough to be rational about anything. Looking back, I cannot even fathom how I did what I did and the pain I caused others. For that I am forever truly sorry. So there I was, on a roller coaster ride of emotions, and I'm up at the top of the hill enjoying things, never seeing that what goes up must come down! And it didn't take long for it to come down. Soon the reality of what I had done set in and the things I would have to face as a result hit home. It took us three days to get to Florida and, once we arrived, it was only a day before we were headed back home. The thought of trying to survive without my family, my only true sense of stability, was terrifying. They were always there for me and now I was taking myself so far from them. Who would be there for me now? This man I ran off with that I truly did not know all that well? I mean, I didn't just meet him, but really how well do you know someone you work with for six months a couple days a week when there isn't much time to interact at the job? I really didn't know too much. Was I banking on that? Not really. I didn't rationally think anything through. A brain unbalanced doesn't really think anything through properly. All I knew was that I didn't want to remain where I was, emotionally-speaking, and I seemed to feel a whole lot better when I was around this man so, there you go. There's my answer! I don't think so. This man was/is not a bad man, but let's be real; this is not a normal occurrence. This is not how it's supposed to be. Maybe in the movies they could pull it off but certainly not in real life. In real life there is hurt and pain and a husband left behind and a wife and child left behind by him. That is not easily handled for anyone unless we were void of any care in the world. We weren't that far gone. So we traveled back, planning to live an hour from our family members so we could be close but not so close that we would be constantly feeling the weight of what we had done. After all, now we would probably be viewed as terrible, horrible people who took off on their spouses – adulterers! Cursed be you!

We made it back from Florida and I phoned my mom. She was so relieved to hear from me after a week of being missing. How terrible a person can you be to do that to your mother? I went to her house and she called my husband. We met at our home. The man I took off with went back to his wife and daughter. I was broken by everything; messed up to say the least. My husband allowed me back in our home because I was clearly not well. He wasn't taking me back necessarily, but we agreed I needed help. So for the first time, I went to a psychologist recommended by his divorce attorney, although he wasn't drawing up papers quite yet – that happened only after further indiscretions. So, I went. I was told I was suffering from clinical depression and I was prescribed an antidepressant, Celexa, along with psychotherapy. We were supposed to go to therapy together at some point but that never happened. What really mattered was that I get help, although I think we should have also gotten help together. So I started right away on the antidepressant. Immediately I began to notice how beautiful the flowers were – life seemed to be a whole lot brighter. This was good! I went to psychotherapy to discuss the ins and outs of my emotions and how I was feeling. The medication, even though it was having its positive effects, was also having other negative effects such as extreme fatigue. I had to take naps during the day and I still had difficulty dealing with things, so I would nap to try to feel better. I decided to start my own business personal training, which was definitely helpful as it was using my knowledge. I obtained a few clients then a few more. The problem was that on this medication I was really tired, so tired that

I fell asleep at the wheel twice. Not good! The positive benefits seemed to wear off, too, so now I was taking a medication that was basically just making me tired and not really helping me. In fact, after a few months I started to feel a whole lot worse but because I had previously been doing better as noted by the psychotherapist, I didn't need as much therapy so I kind of went unnoticed during this time. I started to have all kinds of fluctuations in my emotions but mostly agitation. I would feel agitated one moment then get depressed. I would feel better then worse. A rollercoaster, but one that had highs and lows a whole lot more frequently except I wouldn't say the highs were all that great. Although I do remember a particular moment where I felt on top of the world; this song I loved came on the radio and it triggered me to go into a bout of mania. I felt like I was high on something, although I wasn't. I started driving fast and singing. I felt invincible at that moment. It was the first moment that someone else noticed I wasn't quite right. I noticed it, too. Up until then, my highs were not really highs. I mostly felt low all of the time. However, I still did not go back to the psychotherapist to discuss this with him and continued the medication. It wasn't long before I was so low I couldn't cope with life. It was September 6, 2000. I didn't want to deal with it anymore. I told my husband I was going to kill myself. We were at my parents' house. It was Labor Day. I went to their cabinet, grabbed a bottle of pills, and started walking down the road. I took the bottle of pills and just kept walking. I walked to the end of their road and my mom came by with the car and told me to get in. I said, "No! No one can help me!" and kept walking. She didn't know about the pills. I turned down the next road and kept walking to the end about two miles from my parents' home. My dad came by in his car and got out. He decided to walk with me. We continued to walk around the block (about four miles). He never knew I took any pills. We arrived home and nothing happened. The whole time I was waiting for something to happen.

Not sure what, but something. You don't take a bottle of pills and have nothing happen. At least I didn't think that was possible. Just one of the many times God's angels were watching over me. I clearly see God's hand of protection as I look back on my life. My dad was wonderful that day, just coming along-side me and being there. I'll always remember that.

My husband and I left my parents' house that day. I told my husband what I had done, but was experiencing no effects. We went out and bought a dog, a Rottweiler, and named him Rudy. It was our way of coping with everything going on – a distraction. It wasn't long before I had to say I needed to feel that good feeling again. The one I had felt almost a year before when I had relief from my depressed mind. I sought out the man I had taken off to Florida with. At this point, he was separated from his wife. My husband and I had agreed we would go our separate ways. I was in such turmoil. I was torn in my emotions and in my mind. I wanted to stay. I wanted to leave. I just wanted to feel normal – that is all. I didn't know where I could find that, but clearly it wasn't where I was at, or so I thought. So we agreed that we would separate. Meanwhile, I found this man to give myself a self-prescribed dose of endorphins. It's funny how emotions can impact brain chemistry so strongly. Could someone bottle that please, without any of the side effects that medication brings? Wouldn't that be great? Then we could experience it in life without going to extremes to try to get it.

Back I went to the psychotherapist and I was told that I had been misdiagnosed. I wasn't really suffering from clinical depression but from bipolar disorder. I was really manic-depressive, characteristic of highs and lows, and because I was put on an antidepressant without a mood stabilizer, it caused me to go into "rapid cycles". Now that I was properly diagnosed, I needed to take an antidepressant along with a mood stabilizer and, of course, psychotherapy. I wasn't buying it. I realized the mood disorder thing. I was on a roller-coaster ride much worse after the medication than before. I'll give you that but more medication after what I experienced because of the medication – no thanks! I'd rather not play Russian Roulette with my life. I was told I would not be treated with psychotherapy if I did not take medicine. And if I did not take medicine, it was highly likely that I would commit suicide. There is no cure. Isn't that nice? Thanks for the hope when I was feeling so hopeless. Just to get out of the office, I agreed to take the prescription slip but I never filled it. Thank you Jesus, that I did not! I didn't know that in less than a month I would be pregnant with a child who would change my life. Who knows what that medicine could have done to my son? I decided I would find another way. I would find a cure. I am stubborn like that. I don't accept defeat. I have fight in me. Don't tell me something is impossible. If a cure for bipolar disorder was impossible, then I was believing that it was possible. I did have faith in God and I started to exercise it.

My husband and I parted and I found an apartment. I continued to work with clients in personal training and go from house to house. One morning I had a client early; I think it was a 6 am appointment. On my way to their house, a deer suddenly appeared in front of my car. This thing had huge antlers and all I could envision were them coming straight through the front windshield at me, so I swerved to miss him. I ended up turning around and in the ditch. Immediately the people in the house nearby came running out. They phoned the police. I was shaking. My car was totaled, and I went to the doctor to get checked out. It was at the doctor's that I was asked if I could be pregnant. Not having really thought about, it I realized I could be so they made me pee in a cup. Sure enough, I was. And after the record of attempting to take my life in the file, I was not allowed to leave the doctor's office until I spoke on the phone with a relative and was headed to their house. When I got to this relative's house and told her, let's just say it didn't go over well.

This began the years of judgment from friends, relatives – not all of them, but certainly some. What did I expect after all? No one knew that my brain chemistry was a mess. Everyone thought I was fine. One of my close relatives was puzzled how I could do such a thing. She couldn't understand how I could just take off when I went to Florida and now this. This was NOT how I was raised! I knew better. Don't get me wrong here; I take full responsibility for my actions but the truth is the truth. My brain chemistry was off!

I want to acknowledge that, although some family members were unsupportive and judged me, I had some who were truly wonderful. One of them was my younger sister, Bette, the one I spent most of my childhood with, day in and day out as my best friend. We were close in age, and when she found out about me being missing she went out and bought me a ring. As soon as she knew I was home safe she gave me that ring and that I will never ever forget. She also lived with me a couple months before I gave birth to my son, and then the three weeks after until she was married. She helped me during some of the most difficult times of my life. I can say that all of my siblings now are truly there for me and love me. I also understand that we are all human and that not everyone will understand what you are going through and it's ok. I understand that those who judged me did so because they couldn't relate to my pain or know what I was going through, heck I didn't understand my pain either at the time.

So there I was, in an apartment separated from my husband, alone, and pregnant. I hit rock bottom; my lowest low. I cried out to God, and I surrendered my whole life to him for the first time. I was raised in the church and had accepted Christ into my heart at a young age, but I never fully surrendered my life until that day; that lonely, desperate day. I still did not want to live, but I knew I would never hurt the baby inside me. I hung on for that baby and I let God take over. I told Him that I couldn't live my life, and that He needed to. Whatever He wanted me to do, I would do. That began my transformation of faith. I started to read the Bible multiple times a day. I listened to ministers on TV. I went to every service I could and visited other churches. The message seemed to be the same: 'if only you will have faith'. My faith grew so much I believed that ANYTHING was possible. I believed that God could heal me completely – that I could be healthy, happy, and whole. I stood on that for many years as God brought me the deliverance that I needed. This is the wisdom in the pages ahead. I pray that He blesses and transforms your life as He has mine.

It could have been a radical, immediate transformation but it wasn't. If it had been, I wouldn't have gained the knowledge to help others. Instead, He took me through a process of learning more and more and setting me free – layer by layer. The journey was not always easy, but with the tools He gave me, I had hope; hope that made me want to live, hope that told me there were brighter days ahead, hope that said I'm never going back to where I was, hope that made me realize I need God every moment of every day. I needed a purpose in life and this was it. My purpose was to find a cure. My purpose was to be set free so that I can be a blessing to others and show them the path to freedom.

So here I was alone in that apartment, and sick as a dog with morning sickness. I've never felt such fatigue in my entire life like I felt those first couple months. I could barely get myself off of the couch. Because I had my own business, being sick and tired wasn't working out well for me. I had to cancel so many appointments because I was sick all the time. I wasn't making any money as a result, and thankfully was able to get out of my apartment lease. But where to go? My dad didn't want me to live with them, although my mom would have loved it. So where could I go? To my Aunt Suzie's in Connecticut. She would soon become and still is my rock. She is always there for me no matter what. I love her so much. She helped me to grow in my faith. She is the most wonderful woman you could know. She has a heart of gold and wants to help everyone. She opens her home to so many people in need. She is amazing. I am truly thankful for her love. I lived with her for four months before I decided I needed to go back home to get ready to deliver the baby. I hadn't seen a doctor the first seven months and was planning to just go to the emergency room. As it approached, I got nervous and wanted a doctor so I went back. Because I hadn't seen a doctor, they gave me a delivery date of anywhere from May 15th to July 1st. Well, what do you know? My son, my amazing gift from God, arrived on July 4th. This boy saved my life. He literally saved my life and he has been the most precious treasure ever. I thank the Lord for him every day. The birth of my son began the process of healing for me emotionally. I now had a reason to live. I had the most amazing gift a person can ever be given – a child. That was so overwhelming to me that I would just break down, crying tears of joy. I wasn't alone anymore either. I could take him with me everywhere that I went. He is by far the best thing that has ever happened to me.

Since my brain chemistry seemed to be on a high from the birth of my son, I began my research into foods and the brain. I quickly learned so many things about food and mood, and began to incorporate them immediately. I was determined to find a cure, to not let this disorder beat me up again. It didn't happen overnight, and it turns out there are multiple factors that come in to play, but the journey was well worth it. Anything to be free! Anything to be normal, as long as it didn't have negative consequences. I wasn't going on a wild escapade again – that wasn't the path I was going to take. The path I was on was a Godly path. Mind you, I wasn't perfect along the way. I took a few side roads now and again, but God has always brought me back and made me wiser through it all.

I learned how certain foods affect your mood, the most common being gluten and casein – both of which, it turns out, I had terrible problems with. It helped a lot removing these from my diet initially. I learned how blood sugar plays a huge role in your energy levels and mood. Stable blood sugar is definitely the key to stable energy and mood. I learned how to combine foods to keep my blood sugar and mood stable, how important protein and fats are to the manufacturing of your mood-enhancing brain chemistry, how chemical and/or heavy metal toxicity can hinder brain function, how a healthy gut is needed for a healthy brain, how important hydration is to all our bodily processes, how sleep and the health of the adrenals directly impacts your brain chemistry, how if hormones are off brain chemistry follows, how emotional well-being and being able to handle stress and your thoughts play a major role, and that there's a spiritual battle for your mind and how you can conquer it. I praise the Lord for the abundance of wisdom He has given me.

I am proud to say that I have full confidence in who I am in Christ. I am healthy and happy! I have a sound mind and a love for life. God has set me free from the burden of bipolar disorder. I pray that God leads you to the areas you need help with so that you can be healthy in mind, body, and spirit. That's not the end of my story. You will hear more parts of what God has brought me through throughout this book. He has set me free from so much. Praise be to God!

Chapter 2
Building Optimal Mental Health

In order to obtain total freedom from mental illness, I believe it is important to address five components to healing: spiritual, emotional, neurological, nutritional, and physical fitness. I believe that any one of these addressed separately can only bring you so far. All five areas need to be addressed and maintained on a regular basis in order to obtain true health and freedom from mental illness. There is a specific order to addressing these components. I opted to put spiritual healing first, because with God all things are possible and the road looks a lot brighter when we have faith. Once that has become real to you, then dealing with your thoughts and emotional trauma in your life will set the stage for success when nutrition and fitness are implemented.

Let's compare the building of a house to the building of your mental health. When an individual decides to build a house, he first properly plans out his course, digs the basement, and lays the foundation. Having the plan/vision laid out in advance allows him to envision the end result without trying to skip ahead and put the roof on before the walls are up. That sounds ridiculous when talking about a building, but is what many people will attempt to do in order to build their mental health. This goes for medication as well as supplements to aid mental health. Properly laying the foundation sets the stage for a sound structure that will hold up to the outside elements and protect the integrity of the home. A properly-laid foundation will lead to the ability to provide sound and level floors and walls throughout the rest of the home. If there is a problem on one of the upper floors it is much easier to fix if the root of the problem is not coming from the foundation. If there is a crack in the foundation, this will ultimately impact the rest of the building structure. This problem is much more difficult to solve, and likely will be quite costly. If the foundation is sound then it will be much easier to resolve the problem. Your mental health can be explained in a similar fashion. If the foundations of mental health are not intact, then it is much more difficult to resolve problems. We must first look at the foundations of mental health before we can even consider the health of the walls and floors.

When building sound mental health, it's important to build a solid foundation of spiritual and emotional healing with a strong nervous system to provide the floor base. Once this is established, then nutrition and fitness will be much more effective, and you set the stage to obtain optimal mental health.

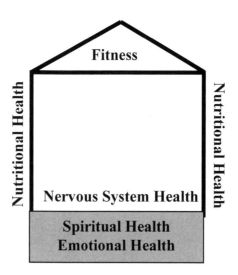

Chapter 3

Building A Healthy Mind Spiritually

I want to begin by saying that I have been brought up in the church and had the opportunity to learn about Christ at a very young age. Not everyone has had that same experience and you may be reading this not having had any experience with religion or God. I want you to know that that's okay. I have found this aspect of my life to be instrumental in helping me mentally and I want to share that with you. I believe that having faith in something bigger than you can be so helpful in building hope, and hope is what we all need in life. Hope helps us to see that the future can be bright. Faith allows us to believe that there is a God who loves us and is looking out for us. This can be beneficial and bring tremendous peace and rest in our minds. I personally believe that it does not matter what religion you are, but it's about a relationship with our Creator. Anyone can have a relationship with God if you desire one. I believe that the power of faith can create a strong foundation for mental health and is why I have put it first.

I cannot be thankful enough for my upbringing to know the Lord Jesus as my Savior. He is my best friend and I promise you if you ask him to be your best friend you will never regret that decision. If you do not know Jesus and you want to know him simply say this prayer:

"Dear God, I ask you to come into my heart. I believe you sent your son Jesus to die on the cross for my sins. I believe he rose from the dead and is seated at the right hand of the Father. I believe in you and that my eternal salvation is secure in you. I ask you to be my best friend. Lead me to the truth and set me free from mental illness." In Jesus' name, Amen

I believe God's word that says if you ask for bread, He won't give you a stone (Matthew 7:9). God wants to give you good things. His plans for your life are good (Jeremiah 29:11). He wishes above all things that you prosper and be in health (3 John 1:2). God is NOT a man that He should lie (Numbers 23:19)! We have all experienced a person in our lives who has lied to us and hurt us. With God we can be safe and know that His promises are true. He wants good for our lives and He wants to prosper us and not harm us. As humans, we make mistakes, it's impossible to be perfect but with God all things are possible (Mark 10:27). You may have been given an incurable diagnosis. You may have been told that you need medication for the rest of your life. You may have been told this is genetic and you need to live with it, just cope to the best of your ability. You may have been told that there is no true and real freedom. I'm here to tell you that God sent His son Jesus to this earth to bring us life and to bring it abundantly. Get ready to live the abundant life!

7 Steps To Building A Strong Spiritual Foundation
Step 1: Develop a relationship with Christ

To build a strong foundation spiritually, you need to begin with a relationship with Jesus Christ. If you do not have a relationship and want one, simply say the prayer at the beginning of this chapter. Then begin the elements described here to develop your relationship with Christ. In order to do that you need to read the Word of God regularly, pray (simply a conversation with God), and begin to experience God's love. This will lead to a strong faith and trust in God that will transform your life and mind. When we truly trust in God and give up control of our lives, we can have peace in the midst of whatever we are going through. Sometimes when life gets difficult, we can have a hard time understanding how God can be in the midst of it. However, we only see a small piece of the puzzle that is in front of us at any given time. God sees the whole picture. We may not always understand what is happening but we can trust God, knowing He sees the end from the beginning. The Lord tells us not to worry about our lives (Matthew 6:25-34), that He will take care of every need. When we truly believe this, life becomes much easier to live.

Step 2: Read the Word of God daily

You will need to have a bible that you can read daily. Many churches will give you a bible if you are a new believer. One thing that has truly transformed me and my mind is memorizing the Word of God. Memorizing God's Word causes you to meditate on it and that is what we are instructed to do in Joshua 1:8, *"Do not let this Book of the law depart from your mouth; meditate on it day and night, so that you may be careful to do everything written in it. Then you will be prosperous and successful."* Who doesn't want to be prosperous and successful? This includes being successful with your health. Start with one verse that inspires you, and continue to speak it and meditate on it. Here is a great verse to start with:

> *"I can do all things through Christ who strengthens me." Philippians 4:13*

This is a scripture that my brother has quoted many times while running and it has always brought him strength. I challenge you to do the same during difficult times. Even if you don't have a bible with you at all times, if the Word is in you then you can meditate on it. I recently memorized Psalm 91 – what an awesome chapter of the bible! There is so much in there. I highly recommend memorizing it. It brings comfort and reminds us of God's promises to us to protect us even when all around us is falling apart. Start with one verse each day and add a verse every day. Continue to repeat it until it's like remembering your birth date. If that's too difficult, start with memorizing one verse per week and then add to it. Trust me, if you do this, it will bring life to you. When I was pregnant, I memorized the entire book of James. I can still quote parts of it 14 years later that continue to remind me of God's goodness.

I want to share a revelation that came to me recently in James. We are directed to ask God if we lack wisdom in James 1:5-8,

"If any of you lacks wisdom, he should ask God, who gives generously to all without finding fault, and it will be given him. But when he asks, he must believe and not doubt, because he who doubts is like a wave of the sea, blown and tossed by the wind. That man should not think he will receive anything from the Lord; he is a double-minded man, unstable in all he does."

We need wisdom in every single area of our lives. This includes wisdom regarding our mental health. God promises to give us wisdom if only we would ask. How many times do we neglect to ask God for wisdom over a situation? How many times do we run to the doctor before seeking God? God has called us to seek Him first in all situations. This is very important when it comes to your mental health. Seek God before going to a psychiatrist or psychologist and allow God to lead you. Although I believe it is important to get professional help, we need wisdom to know where to go. This will make all the difference in the world. God is all-knowing, and when we learn to ask Him to direct us and learn to follow His lead we can remain at peace. If you are unable to trust your mind and thoughts while you are working to heal then go to someone you can trust who can guide you in faith to the help that you need.

Reading a verse from the bible and meditating when we are not feeling well mentally or emotionally can have a huge impact on how we feel. I have often quoted scripture in times of stress or anxiety and it has brought me tremendous peace. I encourage you to find verses in the bible that help you in these times and write them out in a journal or post them around the house.

Here is a verse I have quoted during many difficult times in my life from James 1:12, *"Blessed is the man who perseveres under trial, because when he has stood the test, he will receive the crown of life that God has promised to those who love him."*

Step 3: Pray continuously about everything

Prayer is just a conversation with God. Personalize it and speak to Him whatever is on your mind. He loves you so much more than you know. He cares about everything that you are going through. Reach out to Him. Give Him every worry. Each day continue to cast your cares on the Lord and allow Him to take them from you.

Throughout the day if you can remember to first go to God in prayer, peace will continuously be with you. Pray about everything all the time. You can pray anywhere, even in the middle of a conversation you can pray in your mind. Make God your best friend by talking to Him all the time. He is the best friend you have always wanted, and He will never leave you.

Step 4: Build faith by being around other Christians

There is tremendous power in prayer and joining with other believers in prayer. The word says, *"For where two or three gather in my name, there am I with them"* Matthew 18:20. It's important to get and stay connected with others who share your faith. This will help to build your faith and relationship with Christ. Just like any other relationship you have, if you don't speak to the person, the relationship fades. The same goes for

Christ. What would happen if you spent all day in the house with your spouse and neither one of you talked to each other? How great would your relationship be? The same is true of your relationship with Christ. Treat it as you would any relationship that you want to flourish. Share your heart with Him – He knows it anyway. Talk to Him as you would to your spouse. Talk and listen. You can't have a great relationship with anyone that is a one-sided conversation. Having a relationship with Christ involves both speaking with Him (through prayer) and listening. God speaks to us in many different ways. It could be through His Word, through another person, through a minister, a letter, or a dream. I can personally attest to the many ways God has spoken to me. One thing I have learned is that when you are seeking God for answers on something in life, He almost always confirms the answer in multiple ways. And His answer is always one that brings peace. We are to be led by peace. If you have no peace about a situation, do not move in that direction. Wait for God's direction and move in peace.

In order to truly live a life of freedom from worry and anxiety, we need to build faith. The bible tells us that faith comes by hearing and hearing by the Word of God. In other words, the more we hear God's Word; the more we will believe. That goes for anything in our lives. If we are constantly around negativity, we begin to think and believe negatively. If we are constantly around positivity, we begin to think and believe positively. So, in order to grow our faith in God, we need to saturate our lives with Him. To do that we need to be around others who also have faith in God and to read it through His Word, the Bible. The more you have faith in God, the more you will trust Him with your life. When you can give up control of your life, knowing that a loving God has your back and wants only good for your life, you will begin to see Him guiding you. As you follow His lead, you will find freedom and the answers you were seeking.

> ***"Call to me and I will answer you and tell you great and unsearchable things you do not know." Jeremiah 33:3***

Call on other believers when you are struggling, to help lift you spiritually with their words and prayer. This has done wonders for me in times of need. It helps to have others praying for you. One thing I know is that there is power in prayer. I have had many prayers answered and God has brought me tremendous peace in times of distress when I and others have gone to him in prayer.

Step 5: Trust God with all your heart

When we truly trust God in every area of our lives, then we find true freedom. When you can get to a point where you do not concern yourself with what others think of you, but ONLY with what God thinks of you, you will be free! God did not call us to worry about what everyone else thinks. You are here to fulfill your God-given purposes in life, not someone else's. There will be many people who don't understand your purpose; that is because it is your purpose not theirs. It has taken me years to truly trust in God in all areas of my life, but has been so worth it. People will put you down. That is part of life. However, you have the choice to decide if what they do to you is going to impact your feelings of well-being and self-worth. Only you can choose to allow someone else's actions to impact you. I have a sticky note on my computer with the message, "The power to be happy is within me". When we realize that we have the choice to be happy, then there is always something we can do about it. If happiness is outside of you then you can't control it, but the truth is happiness is within you! Trusting God in all areas of your life is choosing to be happy within you, knowing that a loving God has your best interests at heart.

> *"Whoever trusts in the Lord, happy is he." Proverbs 16:20b*
>
> *"You will keep him in perfect peace, whose mind is stayed on you, because he trusts in you." Isaiah 26:3*

Step 6: Love others

Love must permeate all areas of our lives if we are to truly live free. Love allows us to let go of hurt and forgive others. This is where we find freedom from emotional pain and hurt. Holding on to anger and bitterness does not harm the person who hurt you; it harms you. Let go and let God heal you by allowing love into your heart. This is easier said than done, but there are things you can do to help you along the way as you are healing from trauma. You will learn more about how to do that in the following chapter on Emotional Healing.

Step 7: Practice forgiveness

A heart that can forgive is a heart that can be free. When we are able to forgive others, it frees us. Forgiving someone does not make what they did right, nor does it mean that you have to continue to be hurt by them or allow them into your life. Forgiving others allows you to be free from the pain that they have caused you. Learning to see things from others' perspectives and recognizing that we are all human and we all make mistakes is also quite helpful. It doesn't excuse what the other person has done, but it helps us to let go and let God heal us from the pain that others have caused us. You may never get an apology from the person who hurt you so deeply, but you can make a decision to no longer let it hold you back. Allow yourself to forgive them and be free from the pain. It may not be easy at first, and you may have to repeatedly forgive them as the pain comes back into your mind. Over time, as you forgive and let go and bless them, you will find freedom.

REVIEW: Seven Steps to Building a Solid Spiritual Foundation

1. Develop a relationship with Christ. Talk to Him often and allow Him to speak to you.
2. Read the Word of God daily and meditate on it.
3. Pray continuously about everything.
4. Build Faith by being around other Christians.
5. Trust God with all your heart – do not concern yourself with what everyone else thinks about you but ONLY what God thinks of you.
6. Love Others
7. Practice Forgiveness

Chapter 4

Building A Healthy Mind Emotionally

Let me make one thing perfectly clear: It doesn't matter how well-functioning your brain chemistry is if you are constantly being treated like you are worthless, are abused verbally, physically or sexually, or have had some traumatic event occur. At that point, brain chemistry naturally goes out the window. Granted, the healthier your body and brain are, the less likely you are to go overboard if your emotional situation is ripped apart by another person or situation. Nonetheless, your brain chemistry will change in these situations. So what is the remedy for that? Let's begin by discussing emotional healing and some tools to help you obtain it.

Emotion is defined by www.freedictionary.com as *"a mental state that arises spontaneously rather than through conscious effort and is often accompanied by physiological changes; a feeling: the emotions of joy, sorrow, reverence, hate, and love"*. We all have emotions. Some individuals show emotions more than others, but we are all wired to have emotions. We are created to feel. It's what makes us humans and not robots. It's a gift from God but when emotions cannot be controlled, there are problems. Some people have experienced such trauma in their lives that they have either buried these emotions so deeply they appear to have no emotions, or they wear them on their sleeves and the whole world knows. All of this takes a toll on the body physiologically. These physiological changes in the body result in brain chemistry imbalances. So how do we deal with these emotions in our lives? How do we heal from trauma? How do we stop those moments where a traumatic event is triggered and sets off a whole cascade of hormones in the body? This is real. It does happen. A person can feel perfectly fine one moment and, in the next, the body is triggered to respond with stress hormones causing the brain chemistry to change as a result of a triggered traumatic event. When this occurs it can feel as though you will never be able to conquer this. After all, you can't erase the past. You can't erase the hurt and pain; or can you? Wouldn't that be great? I believe that you can change the wiring in your brain to not set off a cascade of stress hormones when you are reminded of your past trauma but it takes patience and endurance. In this chapter, I will give you what I believe to be keys to conquering the trauma in your life. I am, in no way, claiming to be an expert on trauma although I have experienced these triggers from traumatic events and pain in my life. I believe in a God who can do the impossible and I am believing that if you have experienced a severe trauma in your life that God will lead you to healing. Trust in Him and let Him show you the way. I pray that these keys will be the start to your permanent healing from the trauma that you have experienced in your life.

Key #1: Get it out. Although I don't believe that re-hashing your traumatic event and painful experiences in life over and over again is in any way helpful, I do believe that we need to get it out. We do need to talk to someone about what happened – someone who is supportive and will be able to bring encouragement.

Key #2: Free your mind of it. Once you have gotten it out – release it to God. Although God may use your situation to help bring healing to someone else who has experienced a similar situation, do not dwell or think about the traumatic event. *"As a man thinketh in his heart so is he"* Proverbs 23:7. If you constantly think of the painful event, then you will be in constant pain. Instead, fill your mind with positive thoughts of life and the future. This is something that takes training. Negative thoughts breed more negative thoughts, and positive thoughts breed positive thoughts. However, it seems as though the mind naturally goes to the negative – particularly if it's been there a lot in the past. So, depending on where you are coming from, this may take a bit of time; but be patient.

Key #3: Replace negative thoughts with positive thoughts. Decide to not allow your mind to dwell on a negative thought. You may not be able to prevent the negative thought from entering your mind but you can decide to allow it to stay. Instead, dismiss it and replace it with a positive affirmation.

For example, if your mind quickly says when you look in the mirror, "You're fat!" then tell yourself, "God created me and I'm beautiful. With God's help I am becoming healthier every day!" If your mind tells you, "You are worthless, no one loves you!" then tell yourself, "God loves me! I was created for great things! I have worth! God has great plans in store for me!"

Key #4: Hang around positive people. It's hard to be positive in a negative environment. Choose to minimize your time in negative environments, or eliminate it all together if possible. Find friends who encourage you, build you up, and have a positive outlook on life. Negative friends will ultimately bring you down, no matter how hard you try to remain positive. It's like a contagious disease. If you are around negative people, you will soon become negative. The opposite is also true. It is much easier to remain positive when you are around positive people.

Key #5: Accept failure. Failure is just another step closer to success. Learn from your mistakes instead of beating yourself up. You've heard the saying, "What doesn't kill you makes you stronger", right? This is true only if you allow it to make you stronger. This is a choice. If at first you don't succeed with healing from the trauma in your life – try, try again. You will succeed if you don't give up, and trust me, it will be worth it.

Key #6: Discover who you are. Maybe this should be the first key because it is so important. If you know who you are in Christ, it is so much easier to stay positive and accept the beautiful creation that He made when He made you. You are a child of the Most High God! You were born for greatness! Even if you have been through a lot in your life, God will take the ashes and make them beautiful. He will take the broken pieces of your life and make a masterpiece if you let Him. You can walk around with confidence, holding your head high, knowing that God is taking care of you, that he loves you, and that's all you need. There is freedom in knowing to whom you belong. You may not have had the best earthly mother and father, but your Heavenly Father takes the cake! There couldn't be a better Father!

Two books, *You Can Be Happy No Matter What* by Richard Carlson, and *The 10 Secrets to Success & Inner Peace* by Dr. Wayne Dyer, have both been instrumental in helping me to change the way I think. I have also benefitted from many of Joel Osteen's books. These books, as well as reading the Word of God every day, have helped me to renew my mind and set my thinking in the right direction.

OTHER THINGS TO CONSIDER

Seek Professional Help

We would all do well to seek professional help. This is true of every area of our lives. If your car is not running properly do you try to fix it on your own? No; you take it to a person who specializes in mechanics to investigate the problem and fix it for you. That is their area of expertise. While it is always good to study topics in areas of your life where you can take control, it is also quite beneficial and more productive to seek out professionals who have successfully helped others. Why spend hours and hours trying to study how to conquer your fears or heal from emotionally traumatic events in your life in an attempt to heal yourself, when you can go to someone who has spent a good portion of their life studying and helping others and has experience? I suggest going to your pastor and asking him/her to recommend a good Christian counselor who specializes in healing from emotional trauma. This will help provide you with even more tools regarding your specific situation and accelerate your healing. Be careful here as to who you seek advice from. Always look to God first to direct you.

Being Social for Emotional Health

We were created to be with other people. Some of us may require more socialization than others, but I do believe we all need social interaction for optimal mental health. The bible tells us to not forsake the assembling of ourselves. This means we should not avoid getting together with other believers. This helps to build up our faith and bring encouragement. We all need it!

If you are not involved with others, consider joining a group of other like-minded individuals. It could be a painting class or exercise class, maybe a hiking buddy or prayer group. There are so many things out there to get involved in. If you can't find one, consider starting your own group. You could start a group with others who enjoy crafting or reading. You can choose anything that you enjoy doing.

I find that, if I am alone for too long, my mind starts to wander. I enjoy being alone for short amounts of time, up to a few hours, but not much longer than that. I want to be around people… my family and friends. My husband, on the other hand, likes longer times alone. I think it may be more common in men to like to be alone longer, but everyone is different. For some, social situations cause a lot of anxiety. The right social situations need to be determined for each individual. While getting together with others can cause stress-relief, in the wrong situation, it could cause added stress. The point here is to find a group or simply others to engage with in social interaction on a comfortable level for you that does not cause stress. Some are not good in groups and prefer one-on-one, and that is fine. You will know what you feel most comfortable with. But don't hibernate and isolate yourself from the world. It only leads to the mind constantly thinking and that can lead to trouble. Getting together with others helps get your mind off of just you, and on to other things.

Finding Activities You Love

Whether by yourself or with others it's important to find activities that you love and that provide stress-relief. It could be a walk in the park, getting a massage, reading a book, hanging with friends, going out to dinner, taking an exercise class, doing a puzzle, painting, drawing, dancing, or singing. We all have things that we love to do. I absolutely love to dance! The right music with the right people and I'm having the time of my life. It's like therapy, as it brings life to my body and health to my mind. I also discovered recently that I love to paint! Last year, I painted pictures for all of my nieces and nephews for Christmas. It was so soothing and fun. I also think that we feel good when we are creating things and this was one way to do that. We are created in God's image and he is the Master Creator. I once read that when we are creating, we are closer to our Creator. This sounds right to me. I definitely feel a lot of peace when I am creating things. For you, this could be trying a new recipe or writing a poem. It could be creating a dance step or exercise program. It could be creating a website design or a newspaper article. There are so many things we create in life. Think about what you can create that brings peace and joy to you as you do it. We were not meant to create all things. If it is depleting you of energy and joy, you probably weren't meant to do it.

Explosive Anger

I listened to a talk by Jimmy Evans, of Marriage Today, and he spoke on the topic of explosive anger at a very important moment in my life when I was struggling. He said that explosive anger is a result of not dealing with anger daily, but allowing it to be buried. He believes that it comes from unforgiveness and hurt that is kept inside, and that the scriptures give us the solution to unlocking the pent-up anger that results in us being tormented emotionally and lashing out on our loved ones. It may not even be the ones who have hurt us that we lash out at. Eventually, if you keep anger, hurt, and unforgiveness inside, it will come out and often towards the ones you love even if they had no part in causing it. The solution is found in Luke 6:28, which tells us to *"bless those who curse you, pray for those who mistreat you."* He went on to say that this scripture provides the key to emotional healing: blessing those who curse you! As I prayed on this, God revealed to me that I had harbored unforgiveness toward others who had hurt me, and it was starting to come out and wasn't pretty. So I made a decision to ask God for forgiveness for holding anger and hurt towards these individuals. I forgave them and asked God to forgive me. I then asked God to bless them as I would want to be blessed. Even though I may not have felt like blessing them immediately, I did it anyway. I started to do that for every individual God put on my heart that I had held an offense against. I then began to bless them. Each time a reminder came up as to the hurt someone had caused me, I quickly asked God to forgive me and then bless them. I wasn't perfect, and would occasionally catch myself saying mean things against someone to myself or in my mind, but I immediately recognized it, asked for forgiveness, and then blessed them. The very first time I blessed the people who hurt me, it was more like going through the motions but it wasn't long before I genuinely wanted to bless them. I then noticed that my heart started to completely change toward these individuals, and I was free!

Keeping Your Mind Positive

While reading the book, *The How of Happiness* by Sonja Lyumbomirsky, I learned of a study conducted by University of Pennsylvania professor Martin Seligman and Jeff Levy. The study was conducted on severely depressed individuals. They were directed to log onto a website and recall, then record, three good things that happened each day. After 15 days, 94% of participants experienced relief from severe depression to mild or moderate depression. [1-2] I recommend doing this daily, as it is a great way to keep your mind dwelling on the good things that are happening each day. If you get in the habit of doing this, you will help to keep your mind focused on positive things and moving in a positive, healthy direction.

REVIEW: 6 Keys to Emotional Healing

1. Get it out. Talk to someone who is supportive and who can offer sound advice, but don't continue to re-hash your problems with anyone who will listen. This will only create more anxiety, fear, and/or sadness.
2. Free your mind of it. Release your worries into God's hands.
3. Replace negative thoughts with positive thoughts.
4. Hang around positive people.
5. Accept failure. You are one step closer to success.
6. Discover who you are. You are a child of the Most High God. Walk in confidence with your head held high.

Chapter 5

Building A Healthy Mind Via A Healthy Nervous System

The Nervous System & Mental Health

I was first introduced to the idea that chiropractic care, and specifically the health of the nervous system, could impact mental health when I visited Pro Health, a chiropractic office in Manchester, CT and spoke with Dr. Vasco Valov. I certainly knew that the brain functions via the nervous system, but never recognized the value of a healthy spine and its impact on mental health. This was enlightening to me, as I had been studying mental health, and the various things that impact it, for years. I was educated that cervical vertebral subluxations (misalignment of a vertebra or vertebrae in the neck, which affects your nervous system's ability to communicate) are more apt to be present in individuals with mental health disorders, and the correction of these subluxations could result in improvements in well-being. In fact, Dr. Valov had been in a car accident as a teenager, which negatively impacted his mental health, with which he had had no prior issues. The family was urged by a friend to seek chiropractic care, which dramatically improved his well-being and restored his mental health. The results encouraged him to want to make a career in the field of chiropractic. This prompted me to research chiropractic care and mental health. I came across a study that was conducted on 15 clinically-depressed adults who also had cervical subluxations. The study showed that correction of the cervical vertebral subluxations resulted in a reduction of their symptoms of depression.[1] I also discovered that chiropractic care had specifically been used in the past for mental health disorders. In fact, there were clinics that operated to help alleviate the symptoms of mental anguish. Chiropractic doctor, Gerald Martin Pothoff, witnessed several mentally-ill patients being cured through chiropractic care and, in 1922, he established the first Chiropractic Psychiatric Hospital called Chiropractic Psychopathic Sanitarium, which was later known as Forest Park Sanitarium. In 1926, another chiropractic mental hospital was opened, called Clear View Sanitarium. Both of these facilities were in Davenport, Iowa, but years later the hospitals changed course due largely to economic reasons, and the chiropractic component was removed. [2] Multiple case reports have also been documented that encourage the amazing potential benefits of chiropractic care on mental health. These case studies showed improvements in mental health for depression, anxiety, bipolar disorder, and other mental ailments when spinal corrections were made via chiropractic care. [3-6] If the nervous system is unable to properly function due to vertebral subluxations, then it would certainly make sense that it would impact one's emotional and psychological well-being. The health of the nervous system is an area that should not be overlooked if you want to obtain optimal mental health.

A Healthy Nervous System

The nervous system is how the brain relays messages throughout the body via the nerve pathways. If the communication is disrupted along a nerve pathway, it can cause problems at any point along the nerve path. This is vitally important to the health of the body and brain. The nervous system can be considered the "power" of the body. Just like the power needs to be on in order for your home to have lights and electricity, the body also needs its electrical (nervous) system to be functioning properly in order to be optimally well. This was recently explained to me by chiropractic doctor, Andrew O'Neill (of Coastal Chiropractic & Wellness in Madison, CT). When comparing the nervous system to the electrical system in a home, subluxations can be explained by likening them to a dimmer switch in a room. When you dim the light using the dimmer switch, light is coming through the bulb, but not 100 percent. Subluxations, in a similar fashion, do not allow 100% of nerve impulses to go through, creating dysfunction on the other end. We need our nervous system functioning properly in order for the signals to be properly communicated back and forth from the brain to the rest of the body. If a nerve is being pinched it can affect the function of that body part that is supposed to be receiving the information from the brain that is traveling along the nerve pathway. This can happen when a vertebra is subluxated or when the body is inflamed and causing an impingement of the nerve. Many people have subluxations in their vertebrae as well as inflammation in their body, resulting in less-than-optimal mental and physical wellness. So how do you determine the health of your spine and nervous system?

Chiropractic Care/Physical Therapy

The best way to determine the health of your spine and nervous system is through a chiropractic or physical therapy evaluation. An optimal care plan should include initial evaluations of the spine (x-rays and nerve testing) to determine the current condition of the spine, along with exercises to assist your body in improving spine curvature and care to improve any deviations from normal. Although x-rays have their negative impact they are also very instrumental in identifying what exactly the spine looks like, which is essential to creating a personalized care plan. It should also include periodic evaluations to monitor progress.

I had been to several chiropractors over the years, many of whom never took x-rays to determine the current condition of my spine in order to determine the proper adjustments needed to bring correction. I was also, in the past, not given exercises to strengthen and/or stretch my muscles in order to maintain proper alignment. As a personal trainer, I always questioned this. This kept me from going to any chiropractor on a regular basis, only going when I was in pain, to help bring me back into proper alignment. There were times I walked into the chiropractic office crooked, and walked out straight. It wasn't that I didn't believe they could help, but I never understood why I wasn't being helped more in order to prevent falling back into pain at a later date. This to me was centered in their lack of education to the patient on proper stretches and exercises to maintain a healthy spine curvature. This changed for me when I met a couple of Maximized Living's chiropractic doctors, Dr. Vasco Valov and Dr. Jason Sousa in Manchester, CT. They taught me about the importance of the nervous system, as well as how important it is to not only work to obtain proper spine curvature but also how important the mind, nutrition, fitness, and detoxification is to the process. This was my kind of chiropractic office. I have since learned that there are over 600 chiropractic doctors trained in the Maximized Living way of care, and are helping thousands of people to optimize their health through the five essentials: maximized mind, maximized nerve supply, maximized quality nutrition, maximized oxygen and lean muscle, and minimized toxins.

I am no stranger to back pain. I have spondylolisthesis. You may wonder what that is. Basically, I have a vertebra in my lower back that has shifted forward after an initial fracture of the vertebra. As a result, I need to be very careful with what I do, and am susceptible to sciatica (nerve pain going into my butt and down my legs). Because of this, I need to keep my core (abdomen and lower back) very strong in order to prevent back pain and problems. I recently had the opportunity to meet another one of Maximized Living's chiropractic doctors, Dr. Keith Mirante, with Coastal Chiropractic & Wellness in Madison, CT. Dr. Mirante shared a story of how he was first introduced to chiropractic care at the age of 18. It seems that so many chiropractors have a personal story of how chiropractic care had a dramatic impact on their life and it brought them into the field. Dr. Mirante's story is one I could completely relate to, as he, too, has spondylolisthesis brought on by a sport injury. This injury led to terrible back pain and, ultimately, severe digestive issues. After taking several medications, his father took him to see a chiropractor. He learned that his two problems were one and the same – they both stemmed from subluxations affecting the nerves in his lower back. After working to restore the nerve function through chiropractic care, he was able to get off all medication and return to sports. He ended up working in the chiropractic office where he was helped, and witnessed many miracles just like he had experienced. This resulted in him going on to become a chiropractor himself. This only re-enforces what I spoke of earlier, that your life experiences often lead you to your life purpose.

I believe that it is important to have a properly functioning nervous system in order to obtain optimal physical and mental wellness. So, do all people need to go to a chiropractor to obtain that? I don't believe so. After researching, studying, and praying for God's wisdom regarding this I have come to the conclusion that God did not design our bodies in a manner that we all need to have chiropractic adjustments on a regular basis to function optimally. However, I do believe that there are times when an individual has experienced an injury or trauma to their spine that chiropractic care and/or physical therapy can be absolutely miraculous and instrumental in restoring nerve function. I also believe that there are other things that an individual can and should do in order to maintain proper nerve flow from their brain through their spinal cord to the organs and tissues of the body and that repeated spinal manipulation may not be the best avenue for everyone.

There are potential risks associated with spinal manipulation and I prefer to choose a more conservative approach to restoring and optimizing nerve function on a regular basis. This is a decision that would be dependent upon each individual's personal history and health and one that should be made with prayer and God's wisdom.

Physical Therapy to Restore Nerve Flow

Physical therapy can be a great way to help bring proper alignment to the body and spine after an injury or trauma. I have experienced several occasions that my pelvis was rotated one way or another, usually as a result of playing sports, and it caused my spinal alignment to be affected with subsequent nerve pain. I was extremely blessed to have a very intelligent sister who is not only a physical therapist but a neuro specialist in her field. My sister, Lori, has helped multiple times to bring me back into proper alignment through physical therapy exercises. I can't count the number of times I was in pain, went to her house, and she checked my leg lengths and figured out how to bring me back into alignment by resisting as she pressed on my hip or knee in a particular direction. I can't explain it exactly, but I have to say it worked. I've also brought myself back into alignment with Pilates exercises several times. There are multiple avenues to help the body to restore proper nerve flow.

Physical Therapy and/or chiropractic care are things that some may want to consider particularly if you have had trauma or an injury to your spine and need more assistance to bring the spine back into proper alignment. When it comes to both mental and physical health, the nerves have to be able to communicate with the rest of the body in order for it to function optimally. You will learn later in the book how digestive issues can ultimately lead to mental health issues so it is not just nerve interferences in the neck that could potentially affect brain health but anywhere in the body. Coupling chiropractic care and/or physical therapy with personalized exercises to optimize nerve function can benefit some tremendously in restoring spinal alignment and optimizing the nervous system health. It is always wise to seek God regarding which direction you should take to optimize the health of your nervous system and hence your overall physical and mental health.

Nutrition & Exercise for Nervous System Health

Nutrition and exercise play a role in maintaining a properly functioning nervous system as well. Nutrition helps to keep the organs and muscles functioning in a manner to help maintain nerve flow and keep the body functioning optimally. For example, an imbalance in minerals can result in muscle spasms that can impact spinal curvature and nerve function. Also inflammation in the body can be directly related to nutrition which can impact spinal curvature. Pain in the body from inflammation can cause an individual to favor one side of the body over the other, throw spinal alignment off balance, and thus effect the nervous systems communication in the body. Exercise to achieve and maintain both flexibility and strength in the muscles surrounding the spine is vital to the body's ability to maintain proper spinal alignment. I have found Pilates to be a great exercise in doing just that as it helps to create flexibility and increase strength in the muscles surrounding the spine. I recommend having an exercise specialist and/or physical therapist tailor your program for you based on your needs. For example, having spondylolisthesis, I need to be sure to strengthen my core in a manner as to focus on trunk flexion and minimize extension of my low back, so as to not aggravate my condition. While an individual who has a bulging disc would need to minimize flexion of the spine and focus on extension for optimal results. Having an exercise program created specifically for your needs, based on the health of your spine, is a great way to obtain and maintain proper spinal alignment, and optimize the health of your nervous system and body. I have found that the warm up exercises given to me by the Maximized Living Chiropractic Doctors to increase blood flow and flexibility to the muscles surrounding the spine along with Pilates exercises to strength my core and maintain flexibility in my spine have been instrumental in keeping me out of pain.

Your Nervous System Optimized

In order for your brain to function optimally, the signals from your brain through the nerves and back need to be clearly communicating. That occurs when the nerves are not being impinged upon. Our nerves are designed to give us signals when there is a problem. Pain, as so many of us are familiar with, is a result of nerves being impinged upon. Whether it is from the spine not being properly aligned, or from inflammation in the body pressing on nerves, signals are sent back to the brain indicating a problem, and pain is the alarm system. Many times people will mask these signals with drugs to cover up the pain. That is similar to taking the batteries out of the fire alarm when there is a fire in the house. That is a recipe for disaster. Although it may be very helpful at times in the recovery process to minimize the pain signal, we cannot ignore that it is there and must work to find the root of why the signal is being triggered in the first place. This is especially important if you want to optimize your mental health, as individuals with chronic pain are more apt to be depressed. It's tough to keep a positive mind set when you are constantly in pain, and so you will want to do everything you can to reduce/eliminate pain without compromising health in other areas.

Many communications in the body are made through nerve pathways. Our nervous system is our electrical system designed to direct energy through the body. When this gets disrupted, we can have trouble anywhere in our body, including our brain. Only 10% of the nerve is responsible for indicating pain. As a result, you could have a nerve being affected by a subluxation, and be unaware of it if no pain is present. Any subluxations in the spine will ultimately compromise optimal health. Because of this, it is important to work to keep your spine in proper alignment as designed by God. This occurs by exercising the body to maintain proper alignment, eating in a manner to optimize health in the body, and may also include physical therapy or chiropractic care for some that need additional support in bringing the spine into proper alignment to optimize health.

Chapter 6
Building A Healthy Mind Nutritionally

When it comes to your mental health nutritionally speaking, let's compare it to the building of a house. You must first build strong foundations before you can put up the walls and roof. It is critical that you create a solid foundation first. This you will do by providing an adequate supply of nutrients, building a healthy digestive tract, properly hydrating your cells, maintaining blood sugar stability, and getting sound, restorative sleep. Once this is established, you are ready to work on creating stable floors and walls. In order to do this nutritionally for your mental health, you will work to optimize liver function, bring harmony to your hormones as well as deal with toxicity in your body. Lastly, you will work to put on a protective roof with healthy neurotransmitters, by supplying the body with any additional nutrient support it needs in order to bring balance.

Dr. Abram Hoffer was one of the founders of the field of orthomolecular medicine. Along with other researchers, he discovered that high doses of Niacin and Vitamin C were beneficial for those suffering from schizophrenia. He has written several books one of which is *Orthomolecular Treatment for Schizophrenia: Megavitamin supplements and nutritional strategies for healing and recovery*. I read this book several years ago, and it opened my eyes to the need for super nutrition in the treatment of mental illness. I can say that, for many years, as I was studying to heal myself, I would often feel as though I needed to be hooked up to an IV of high-dose nutrients. The two things that I knew instinctively were that I was toxic and I needed nutrition. In this book, Hoffer speaks of schizophrenia as not one disease, but a group of diseases, and that several factors result in the symptoms of schizophrenia. Some of those factors include nutrient deficiencies, cerebral allergies, and toxic reactions to heavy metals or drugs.[1] He shares many testimonies of lives being radically transformed by treating these specific things. I believe that identifying which factors are impacting an individual is absolutely vital for them to find freedom from the torment of mental illnesses such as schizophrenia and bipolar disorder. The methods laid out here to build the foundations in supplying and optimizing nutrients to the body through a high nutrient diet, identifying digestive problems and food sensitivities (which can result in cerebral allergies), sets the stage to help detox the body and bring balance to blood sugar, hormones, and brain chemistry.

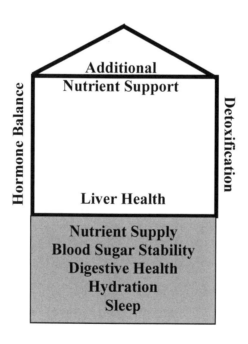

Laying the Nutritional Foundation

As already explained, laying a nutritional foundation is vital to the health of the mind and body. It is important to create a solid nutritional foundation in order to obtain optimal mental health.

- **Nutrient Supply** – Your nutrient supply will come largely from the foods you are eating. For this reason, you want to choose nutrient-dense foods that will nourish and supply the raw materials needed to build your body and brain. Your brain needs a certain supply of nutrients in order to function at its best. The Optimal Mental Health Nutrition Plan will provide the necessary nutrients in order to accomplish this. It is also important to choose healthy food sources that are not laden with pesticides, hormones, antibiotics, or other toxins that will hinder your progress in obtaining optimal mental health.

- **Digestive Health** – The digestive tract includes the entire course that food takes through the body, from entering the mouth until it exits the body through the anus. This includes the mouth, esophagus, stomach, small intestine, liver, gallbladder, pancreas, large intestine, appendix, and rectum. Each part plays a role in the overall health of the digestive tract, and needs to be functioning properly. The digestive tract is where food is broken down and nutrients absorbed into the blood stream and ushered throughout the body where needed, including the brain. The brain needs to obtain nutrients from food in order to function optimally. If the digestive system is not properly functioning then the body and brain will not be getting the proper nutrient supply in order to operate at its best. A healthy digestive tract also includes having a healthy gut microbiome.

- **Hydration** – Water helps to usher nutrients throughout the body and brain as well as remove toxins, both of which are important for overall mental health.

- **Blood Sugar Stability** – If your blood sugar is not stable and you are on a roller coaster ride with your blood sugar levels, then your energy as well as your mood will be riding right along with it. It is vital to your overall health and well-being to obtain blood sugar stability. Mood instability can result simply from the inability of the body to properly balance blood sugar. This is greatly impacted by the diet, and is also impacted by the health of the digestive system. This is not addressed as a separate topic but is incorporated into the Base Dietary Plan that is designed to balance blood sugar.

- **Sleep** – Sleep is vital to your well-being. Lack of sleep will affect your hormones, which will ultimately affect your brain chemistry. While you sleep, your digestive system is allowed to rest and the body works to restore itself and also eliminate toxins. All of this is important to your mental health. By following the Optimal Mental Health Nutrition Plan, you will help to encourage sound sleep. If after four weeks on the nutrition plan you are still not sleeping well, you will be given additional guidelines to help improve your sleep. Sleep is considered a nutritional foundation, simply because nutrition impacts your body's ability to rest. You will learn how different foods impact sleep. There are root issues to the inability to get proper rest. It is in discovering these root issues and correcting them that your overall health and well-being will be optimized.

These five nutritional foundations to mental health are intertwined. The nutrient supply provided by the diet impacts the health of the digestive system, as well as blood sugar stability. Hydration impacts the ability of the body to usher the nutrients supplied from the diet, as well as aid digestion. And a lack of sleep will require a larger nutrient supply, and doesn't allow the digestive system to properly rest and restore.

Creating Stable Floors and Walls

In order to create stable floors and walls in your overall building of mental health you will need to first optimize liver health to then set the stage to create hormonal harmony in the body and deal with toxicity. If you have a strong foundation, and the liver is functioning well, then hormonal imbalances and toxicity in the body will be much easier to resolve. Trying to solve these problems without first laying the nutritional foundations will be similar to banging your head against a wall, expecting to stop the headache. In other words, you won't get far. You may find some temporary relief at times but it likely will not be lasting, and you may cause more damage than before. This is especially true for toxicity. If you do not have solid foundations, and you attempt to detox your body, you will ultimately make your body and mind more toxic. Please do not attempt to do this without first creating a strong nutritional foundation.

> **Liver Health** – The liver is responsible for many things within the body including cleansing the blood and filtering toxins as well as laying the groundwork to manufacture healthy hormones and maintain hormonal balance. It is extremely important that the liver is being well nourished so that it is able to set the stage for hormone balance within the body as well as aid the detoxification processes in the

body in order to maintain optimal mental and physical health.

➢ **Hormonal Balance** – If your hormones are out of balance it will impact the proper balance of your neurotransmitters and thus your mental health. Addressing hormonal imbalances will be much easier once you have stable foundations and floors. An important component to helping recover hormonal balance is to identify the weak link. Your hormones work on a feedback loop, from your brain to your organs and back. The organs relay messages to the brain, signaling when there is not enough of a certain hormone or too much of a hormone and the brain responds by adjusting the signal to increase or reduce the hormone as needed in order to keep proper balance. This occurs through chemical messengers (hormones) in the blood. To get a bit more technical, the hypothalamus relays messages to the pituitary gland, which then relays messages to organs in the body such as the thyroid, adrenals, ovaries, and testes. The organs provide input back to the pituitary with regards to the output of hormones. The pituitary relays the message to the hypothalamus, which then gives the signal to increase those hormones that are needed and decrease those that are in excess in order to maintain a proper balance at all times. Sometimes it is as simple as fixing the communication between the hypothalamus and pituitary. Other times, the organs need specific nutrient support in order to restore proper function. Either way, when the foundations are solid and the body is getting adequate nutrition to supply the hormones, fixing a hormonal imbalance becomes a lot easier.

➢ **Toxicity** – The brain is impacted by the toxicity of the body. We are surrounded by toxins on a daily basis, from pesticides in our food, air, and water to heavy metals from dental work, air pollution and water contamination, from toxic cleaners in our homes to electromagnetic radiation. It's important to minimize your exposure to toxins as much as possible in order to optimize your success. If your nutritional foundations are solid, you will be better equipped to handle toxins when you are exposed to them. Attempting to remove toxins from the body without a proper solid foundation is counterproductive and will likely lead to more toxicity in the body. Do not be too eager to address this area until your body is ready. Your body and brain will thank you if you can be patient in dealing with toxicity.

Protective Roofing

Once you have laid a solid foundation and created stable floors and walls, then you are ready to put the roof on. You may find that having a solid foundation, walls, and floors is all you need to feel good and obtain optimal mental health. If, however, you are still struggling to maintain balanced brain chemistry, then you will want to attack it specifically with additional nutrient support. Many individuals have benefitted from adding specific amino acids into their program in order to optimize mental health. However, I do not recommend trying to determine which amino acids will benefit you without first consulting a specialist in the field. While some people, with less-than-optimal brain chemistry, have benefitted from specific amino acid supplementation, individuals with bipolar disorder, schizophrenia, or other mental illnesses may respond negatively to amino acid supplementation.[2] You may also need certain nutrients which can be determined through deficiency symptoms and/or testing.

Overview
Optimal Mental Health Nutrition Plan

Providing the body with the proper nutrients needed to manufacture your neurotransmitters is essential for optimizing mental health. Nutrition to optimize digestion is also a critical component. This information is provided in detail. The Optimal Mental Health Nutrition Plan is broken down into five phases to make things simpler and allow the body to transition smoothly.

Phase 1
Introduction to the Base Dietary Plan for Mental Health. You will also determine the health of your digestive system and begin work to optimize digestion. You will focus on hydration, blood sugar stability, and will include supplements (to aid digestion and fish oil). Phase 1 lasts for a minimum of four weeks.

- Step 1: Nutrition Foundation - *Nutrient Supply, Blood Sugar Stability (Base Dietary Plan)*
- Step 2: Nutrition Foundation -*Digestive Health*
- Step 3: Nutrition Foundation - *Hydration*

Phase 2
Nutrition Foundation: *Microbiome (Digestive Health) and Sleep Health.* You will continue everything from Phase 1 and begin to include fermented/cultured foods and bone broths by slowly adding them to your diet. Phase 2 lasts for four weeks. You will also determine sleep health and work to improve it.

Phase 3

Floor: *Liver Health.* You will continue what you have been doing in Phases 1 and 2. You will learn how to eat to nourish the liver and support this extremely vital organ to the body in order to set the stage for efficient detoxification in the body. Phase 3 lasts for a minimum of four weeks.

Phase 4

Walls: *Hormonal Balance & Toxicity.* You will continue working on all the things from Phases 1, 2, and 3. You will then identify hormonal imbalances and potentially include supplements to optimize success in correcting imbalances. You will also determine toxicity in the body and begin detoxification through homeopathic supplementation and/or other methods (detox baths, wraps, exercise, dry skin brushing, etc.). Phase 4 lasts for a minimum of eight weeks. The dietary program is designed to help the body to naturally cleanse itself from toxins when all body systems are properly functioning. You will want to incorporate methods to enhance detoxification on a regular basis.

Phase 5

Roof: *Additional Nutrient Support.* Continue Phases 1, 2, and 3 of dietary plan. Continue Phase 4 as needed. If mental health is still not functioning optimally, then a specific nutrient supplement protocol should be determined based on deficiency symptoms and/or testing. I recommend seeking help from a qualified Nutritional Practitioner or Naturopathic Physician in order to determine nutrient deficiencies. Phase 5 lasts as long as necessary in order to bring complete recovery and until the individual reaches optimal mental health.

Review of Optimal Mental Health Plan

Phase	Step	What is addressed?	Length of time
1	1	Base Dietary Plan (Nutrient Supply, Blood Sugar Stability, Removal of Food Allergens)	4+ weeks
1	2	Digestive Health	
1	3	Hydration	
2	1	Microbiome	4+ weeks
2	2	Sleep	
3		Liver Health	4+ weeks
4	1	Hormonal Balance	8+ weeks
4	2	Toxicity	
5		Additional Nutrient Support	varies if needed

Chapter 7
Optimal Mental Health Nutrition Plan

Phase One (4+ weeks)

Step 1: Nutrient Supply

"It is my firm conviction that diet – both what it may be deficient in as well as its potential toxicity – can cause what we label as mental illness." Dr. Kelly Brogan, M.D. [1]

Every person who chooses to make dietary changes or begin taking supplements is responsible for contacting their physician with these changes. This advice does not substitute for the advice of a physician and each person who chooses to follow this program does so at their own risk.

The first step to creating a solid nutritional foundation for overall mental health is to supply the body with adequate amounts of nutrients through the diet. The Optimal Mental Health Nutrition Plan will provide the body with the necessary nutrients to manufacture your brain chemistry and optimize mental health.

Explanation of the Base Dietary Plan: It is important that you fuel your body with lots of nutrient-rich foods in order to have the raw materials needed to manufacture your mood-enhancing brain chemistry. In order to do this, it is important to eat a variety of vegetables and fruits as well as high-quality protein and healthy fats. The health of the digestive tract is also a key component. You need to be able to digest the food you are eating in order to get the benefits of those foods. So relax when you eat and chew your food well. Also take your digestive supplements (more information on this later) to assist the body. Some of you will need more work than others with this. It's important to identify the health of your digestive tract currently so that you can work to improve upon it.

This dietary plan is based on eating three meals per day while eating snacks between meals to keep blood sugar stable. This is important in order to keep energy levels up and your mood stable. Snacks should be fruit. If you are still hungry after the fruit, any allowed protein and/or fat may be included for your snack as well.

Base Dietary Plan

(There is a full list of allowed foods in the following chapter)

Adequate Protein: In order to manufacture your mood-enhancing neurotransmitters, you need an adequate supply of amino acids that come from protein foods. You will be eating a ***minimum of three servings per day*** of healthy proteins. Each serving should be 20-25 grams. Examples of healthy protein sources include pastured or free-range eggs (preferably from a local farm), grass-fed beef, organic free-range poultry, lamb, venison, bison, etc. One serving equates to roughly two to three medium/large eggs, ¼ lb. burger, or a chicken breast the size of an average palm. This does not have to be exact. Listen to your body. It is important to get protein to fuel your brain but it may take some time as you work on your digestive tract, so that you are able to break down the protein. If you do not feel well when you eat protein you are likely having difficulty properly digesting your proteins. If this is the case, you will want to assist your body with a supplement that contains both hydrochloric acid and multiple enzymes, or choose foods to assist stomach acid production. To increase your stomach acid through your diet, you can opt to do one of the following at the beginning of your meal: take apple cider vinegar, digestive bitters, or drink lemon water. Taking a supplement, however, can be an easier method when on the go, and can help to restore stomach acid levels more quickly. Supplementation is not something that you will need to do forever. As you incorporate the guidelines to assist digestion, it will trigger your body to produce proper stomach acid, and you will eventually reduce and eliminate supplementation, as it will no longer be necessary. There is more information on why your stomach needs acid in the digestion section. If you find that your body needs more protein than the three servings, you can add protein in with your snacks throughout the day, but be sure to wait a minimum of 20 minutes after eating your fruit in order to optimize digestion (this is explained further in the section on digestion).

Healthy Fats: Healthy fats are absolutely vital to your brain. You want to have a *minimum of three servings per day* of healthy fats. Examples of healthy fats include avocados, extra virgin olive oil, coconut oil, organic butter (if not sensitive to lactose), and natural fats from healthy meat, eggs, and fish sources. Listen to your body. You do not have to measure here. You need to simply get healthy fats at least three times each day. If you want more of the healthy fats, they are allowed as long as you are not experiencing gallbladder dysfunction. If you lack a gallbladder or are experiencing gallbladder dysfunction (information will be given in the digestion section as to how to determine this), you will need to limit the amount of fat each time you eat and will want to take a supplement to assist the body in digesting the fat (more on that later as well).

Vegetables: You will be eating a *minimum of three servings per day*. Choose a variety of different vegetables, preferably organic, local, and in-season. If not local, choose frozen organic.

Fruits: You will be having _**two servings of fruit per day**_. Choose a variety of different fruits preferably organic, local, and in-season. If not local, choose frozen organic – great for making smoothies. Fruit should be eaten for your snack and not combined with protein and fat, as it can interfere with proper digestion.

Beans: These are allowed but not required on the program. Some individuals may not do well with beans, and should keep them out of the diet particularly while working to heal the digestive tract.

Water: Work up to half your weight in fluid ounces per day, not exceeding 100 fl. oz. Drink filtered clean water; not from plastic. Store water in glass or stainless steel.

Supplements: You should consult with your physician (preferably a naturopathic physician who is educated in supplements) regarding any supplement and prescription medication interactions. See section on the health of your digestive system for more information on supplements.

- **Fish Oil: 3-6 grams/day.** Fish oil has been shown to be very effective in treating depression[2] and can positively impact mental health. Studies have shown that supplementing with omega-3 fatty acids is also beneficial for combating anxiety, ADHD, and bipolar disorder.[3] I do not recommend buying just any fish oil, as many brands have been shown to contain lead and be rancid – both of which will not help your mental health. You should keep your fish oil in the refrigerator to prevent it from going rancid. Here are the professional lines I recommend: Biotics Biomega-3 or Green Pastures Fermented Cod Liver Oil. It's important to note that fish oil is a natural blood thinner. If you are currently taking a blood thinner, then you should consult with your physician prior to taking fish oil.

MY STORY:

Along my journey of discovering how different foods made me feel, I was doing very well when I made a poor decision to drink alcohol in excess on two occasions, one week apart. As I stated earlier, I have never been one to drink much. Alcohol, like sugar, depletes the body of nutrients. This was enough to throw me back in my progress, and send me into a depression that lasted for three months. It was at this point that I seriously considered trying medication again because I was struggling to get myself out of the depression. It was affecting my ability to work, and I went to my parents' house and told them how I was feeling. I even scheduled an appointment with a psychiatrist. Thankfully the psychiatrist could not see me for two weeks. Immediately my father started researching and found information on a Harvard study with fish oil and bipolar disorder.[2] That day I began taking six grams of fish oil per day. In a matter of two days, I was out of the depression that I had been in for three months. If I have recommended one supplement more than any other, it is fish oil for this very reason. For many years I took three to six grams of fish oil per day. It wasn't until I was able to heal my digestive tract that I was able to reduce the amount of fish oil that I took. I also began to include healthy omega-3 fats in my diet where it was severely lacking before, as I hated all seafood growing up. I am very thankful to my father for the wisdom that day. I did go to the psychiatrist two weeks later and I felt wonderful. After all, I had come out of a deep depression that I was in for three months - who wouldn't feel great after that? I was told that I was hypomanic, and that I needed to be on a medication right away to prevent me from going into a full-blown mania and that I also needed to be on a medication long-term. I told the psychiatrist about the fish oil, but she didn't want to hear anything about it. I told her I felt great, that I wasn't hypomanic, and that I just felt wonderful because I was no longer depressed. I also asked her if she had any information on the medication that she was recommending that I take. She said, "Yes, but I highly recommend that you don't read it because if you do you won't want to take it." Wow! That was absolutely correct! I did read it and I did not want to take it and so I didn't. I left her office and I never went back. I never went into a full-blown mania, but I did remain overjoyed at no longer being depressed. I am so glad that I did not take the psychiatrist's advice that day.

☐ **Digestive Supplements.** Supplements to aide digestion such as betaine hydrochloride, multiple enzymes, ox bile (for those without a gallbladder), and a supplement to thin bile for those with gallbladder dysfunction can help to improve digestion much more quickly than without them. You will be determining which ones will be best for you in the section on digestive health.

BASIC DIETARY PLAN REVIEW
✓ Eat **3 meals** per day and **2 snacks**
✓ Meals should contain **20-25 grams of healthy protein**, unlimited healthy fats (depending on ability to digest them), and vegetables
✓ Snacks are fruit
✓ Additional protein and fat can be eaten 20 minutes following your snack if you are still hungry
✓ Occasional beans and/or rice can be included in your diet in small quantities
✓ Adequate **clean water** is important for mental health

- ✓ Supplements should be included to optimize mental health
    - Fish Oil: **3-6 grams/day** taken throughout the day with meals
    - Digestive Supplements: You will learn which digestive supplements are best for you in the section on digestive health.
- ✓ Guidelines to reducing gluten/casein/sugar/artificial sweeteners will be given in the following section. It's important to remove these from the diet gradually to minimize the withdrawal effect.

Removing Common Food Allergens

My Story: I had determined that bread was a problem for me, and so I removed it from my diet for two years before I figured out it was the gluten in foods that was causing me so many digestive, energy, physical and mental health problems. Some of my symptoms included becoming extremely fatigued after consuming gluten, stomach bloating and pain, depression, anxiety, and mood changes. I also had terrible nightmares that seemed to clear up after removing gluten, along with my acne that I had been battling since I was a teen. I had a pretty healthy, clean diet but did not realize that my salad dressing and my marinade contained gluten, and when I finally removed these things, along with other foods I was sensitive to from my diet, my physical and mental health improved dramatically. During this time, I did not have health insurance and so I did not get tested for gluten sensitivity or celiac disease. However, about a year after I had been gluten-free I had a blood test for gluten sensitivity that tested for alpha gliadin. Because I was not consuming gluten at the time, I ate a small square of bread, about the amount you would receive during communion, so that it could possibly show a reaction if I were to have one. I tested positive to the antibodies even with this small *amount of gluten eaten. I did not go on to get fully tested for celiac disease, as I did not see the purpose in it. I clearly had a problem with gluten, and so I have continued to largely keep gluten out of my diet and feel well. After doing much work to heal my digestive system, even if I consume gluten from time to time, I do not have the severe reaction that I used to, either physically or mentally.*

On the Optimal Mental Health Nutrition Plan you will need to remove certain foods, some for a period of time, others possibly permanently. This is important to your success in obtaining optimal mental health. Foods have the ability to break you both physically and mentally if you have an allergy or sensitivity to them. For this reason and to optimize success, I recommend that you remove the most common food allergens from your diet that are likely to cause digestive trouble and mental health problems. You will want to remove wheat/gluten, casein (protein part of milk so this includes milk, yogurt, cheese, and ice cream), nuts (all), corn, and soy. Some individuals who are currently consuming a lot of gluten and casein will want to gradually reduce these in their diet in order to minimize the withdrawal effect. There are charts to assist you in doing this later in this chapter. It's important to also note that eggs are problematic for many as well. I did not exclude them from the program because they contain a lot of good nutrients for the brain. If you have trouble with eggs, then eliminate them as well. This goes for any foods that you have a known sensitivity to. We are all different, so you may have trouble with foods that are not on this list.

Gluten and Casein Intolerance

"Whether we look at depression, anxiety, or behavioral problems, such psychiatric symptoms are often eliminated by the simple removal of gluten from the diet." James Braley, M.D., and Ron Hoggan, M.A. Dangerous Grains [10]

Gluten is a composite of proteins (gliadin and glutenin) found in wheat, rye, barley, spelt, kamut, and bulgar. Gluten, from the latin "glue", is hidden in many foods, as it helps to bind foods together. Because of this you will often not find the word 'gluten' listed in the ingredients even if it is present. Some things that gluten can be hidden in are condiments, salad dressings, marinades, and spices. As defined by webmd.com, *"Celiac disease - also known as celiac sprue or gluten-sensitive enteropathy -- is a digestive and autoimmune disorder that results in damage to the lining of the small intestine when foods with gluten are eaten."* [4] Individuals with celiac disease cannot consume gluten without damaging effects. However, many individuals who do not have celiac disease can be sensitive to gluten, even if their blood test is negative for gluten sensitivity. One of the challenges to the standard test for sensitivity is that they often only test for antibodies to alpha gliadin and not the other gluten proteins. Also, if an individual has removed gluten from their diet and then takes the test, they will be less likely to have a reaction with antibodies in their blood since the offender (gluten) has not been consumed recently. Gluten needs to be in the diet when the test is administered for highest accuracy. However, it may still not detect sensitivity even when one is present, since the test is not measuring all gluten proteins. Dr. David Perlmutter, author of *Grain Brain*, recommends the Cyrex Labs, Cyrex Array 3 test for a more comprehensive marker for gluten sensitivity.[5] I have personally worked with several individuals who had a negative blood test for the standard gluten sensitivity (testing antibodies to alpha gliadin) who clearly did not do well on gluten. I have witnessed many miraculous health changes in individuals who have removed gluten from their diet who were sensitive (with or without a test to prove it) including improvements in mental health, energy, arthritis, MS, fibromyalgia, skin conditions (acne, psoriasis, eczema), headaches, erectile dysfunction, and more.

Much research has been done to link gluten's potential direct and indirect impact on the brain and mental health. Many studies have linked mental health problems to gluten sensitivity and/or celiac disease including anxiety, depression, mood disorders, ADHD, autism, and schizophrenia.[6] For this reason, it is very important to remove gluten from your diet for at least four weeks in order to identify if you are sensitive to it. There are other methods to determine sensitivity apart from blood testing for antibodies. One of the best methods is the elimination diet. On this program, you are doing just that by removing the most common food allergens out of the diet. After a minimum of two weeks of not having these foods in your diet, you should notice some changes in how you feel. With the allergy elimination diet you then would re-introduce one food at a time to test for a reaction. Because you have had the food out of your diet, you will likely react more strongly. This verifies the sensitivity. You may have sensitivity to more foods than are on this list. I was sensitive to multiple foods that I can now eat without problems. By keeping these foods out of your diet while you work to heal your digestive tract, you will have the most success. Once the digestive tract is healed, you may be able to re-introduce some of these foods. However, for some of you, you will need to keep gluten and casein out of your diet permanently to optimize your mental health. Let me give you a little more information as to why gluten and casein can be so problematic for some.

Casein is a protein found in milk, cheese, yogurt, ice cream, and other milk products. Both gluten and casein can have a detrimental impact on mental health in certain individuals. Many individuals with autism, bipolar disorder, and depression have benefitted from both a gluten- and casein-free diet. A study conducted on 471 participants (207 non-psychiatric; 264 bipolar) tested for the presence of antibodies (Anti-Saccharomyces Cerevisiae Antibodies

ASCA marker for inflammatory bowel disease) in the blood for dietary proteins including gluten and casein. The studies showed that the bipolar group had significantly higher levels of antibodies to proteins tested with a 3.5-4.4 fold increase odds ratio for disease association.[7] Other studies have shown increased antibodies to casein in some individuals with schizophrenia, and one study in particular showed a seven to eight fold increase when compared with non-psychiatric controls.[8] This is significant, and one should consider the potential impact that dietary changes of removing these stressors (gluten and casein) can have on overall physical and mental health.

Gluten and casein can also act as opiates and have a drug-like effect on certain individuals who are unable to properly digest these proteins.[9] This impact can cause what is called an allergy addiction, where an individual is addicted to the food that they are allergic or sensitive to. This can make it difficult when you try to remove these foods. Ron Hoggan, author of *Dangerous Grains,* explains this in his book:

"The addictive nature of gluten is often overlooked. For some, the first days and weeks of following a gluten-free diet are characterized by food cravings, disorientation, irritability, sleepiness, depression, mental fogginess, fatigue, and/or shortness of breath. If you are a member of this group, the very fact that you are experiencing many of these symptoms should reinforce the need to exclude gluten from your diet. These are common symptoms of withdrawal of detoxification from gluten-derived opioid and brain neurochemical imbalances. The evidence suggests that about 70 percent of celiac patients will experience these symptoms when beginning a strict gluten-free diet." [10]

These symptoms can occur if you have a gluten and/or casein sensitivity and something you need to be aware of. To avoid these withdrawal symptoms and potential mental breakdown in the process of eliminating these foods you may need to gradually reduce these in your diet until you are no longer consuming them. This will lengthen the time you stay in Phase One of the Optimal Mental Health Plan. You will want to follow all the dietary guidelines spelled out here, with the exception of gradually reducing your casein/gluten over the first four weeks. Once completely out of your diet, you will continue the dietary plan for an additional four weeks before moving on to Phase Two. This is beneficial by gradually making the changes throughout the program in order to optimize your success in the long run. I can tell you from personal experience and work with many clients, that trying to make too many changes all at once can be detrimental to mental health and can result in aborting the program altogether. You will want to minimize that by easing into the program. If you find that you have more than four to five servings of gluten and casein in your diet each day, then you will want to reduce them gradually by following the chart on the following page. By doing this you will help to ease the withdrawal reaction, but you will also be delaying feeling better overall, so keep that in mind and focus on the end goal. Once gluten and casein are completely out of your diet, you should start to feel a lot better. This is the beginning of the journey and you will need to continue to supply your body with lots of nutrient-rich foods to manufacture your brain chemistry, as well as continue to move forward in the program by working on each component until you reach optimal mental health.

To determine how many servings of gluten or casein you are consuming each day consider the potential sources here:

- Gluten Grains: wheat, barley, rye, semolina, spelt, kamut, bulgar
- Foods that often contain gluten: crackers, pasta, muffins, cakes, pastries, cereal, cookies, gravy, dressings, sauces, beer, oats (oats are often cross-contaminated in processing)
- Casein: milk, cream, sour cream, cheese, yogurt, ice cream, and any other milk products. Some individuals can tolerate goat's milk, as it is a different form of casein.

Keep in mind, gluten is hidden in many things so you may be consuming a lot more than you think you are.

If you currently have four or more servings of gluten and casein in your diet daily, you will want to reduce by the following chart to minimize the withdrawal effect. As was already mentioned, gluten and casein can have a drug-like effect on the brain, and so the possibility of withdrawal symptoms should not be taken lightly. Please gradually reduce this to minimize the withdrawal effect and maximize your ability to maintain the diet over the long run.

Program to Reduce Gluten/Casein Gradually	
Week 1	4 Servings/Day
Week 2	3 Servings/Day
Week 3	2 Servings/Day
Week 4	1 Serving/Day
Week 5	0 Servings/Day

If you currently have more than five servings of gluten and casein in your diet per day, then you will want to determine how many servings you currently have and create a program to reduce them gradually by one to two daily servings per week.

This may be the most difficult part of the program. However, if you are following the base dietary plan, you will be getting plenty of foods to keep you full and satisfied. After a short while you will not miss these foods especially when you are feeling in a better mood. This does not mean that these foods will necessarily need to be kept out of the diet forever. Keep them out for at least four weeks and see how you feel. You should be able to add some of them back into your diet in the future. You will, however, want to add the proper sources. For example, with milk, you will want to find a healthy raw source if you are able, to add this back into your diet in the future. Go to *www.realmilk.com* to find a local supplier of raw milk. For now, let's keep it out of the diet. I do not recommend adding gluten back into your diet on a regular basis, even when you have gone through all the phases and are feeling mentally well. Soy impacts hormones and can wreak havoc. When hormones are affected, brain chemistry is affected. Please keep this out as well. Nuts and corn are difficult to digest, and can cause aggravation to the lining of the digestive tract as well as inflammation in the digestive tract if there is a sensitivity. Please keep these foods out while you work to restore the health of your digestive system. You may be able to re-introduce these foods in the future but it may take some time.

Here is a list of foods to remove from your diet in order to optimize mental health:

- Wheat/Gluten
- Milk/Casein (not butter unless lactose intolerant)
- Nuts
- Soy
- Corn
- Any other known food you have a sensitivity to

Sugar Addiction & Withdrawal

Sugar acts like Pac Man, eating up nutrients that the body needs to manufacture brain chemicals. To maximize nutrition to the brain, you will want to reduce/eliminate sugar in your diet. Sugar is addictive, and so removing it can be difficult. Similar to gluten and casein, individuals who have a lot of sugar in their diet will likely experience withdrawal symptoms if sugar is completely eliminated all at once. These symptoms can include fatigue, headaches, anxiety, irritability, depression, moodiness, and more. Because this can negatively impact mental health you will want to slowly reduce sugar in your diet to avoid these problems. Follow the chart on the following page to gradually reduce the amount of sugars/starches that you have in your diet currently. Consider this list of sugars/starches to help you determine how many you currently have in your diet.

Sugar and High-Glycemic Starches (15-20 grams per serving): candies, chocolate, doughnuts, gummies, mints, cookies, cakes, pastries, pasta, bread, etc. I am not including all starches in this list, just high-glycemic processed foods.

A study involving 3,000 participants concluded a higher incidence of depression among those who ate more processed foods than those who ate more whole foods.[11] It is very important to greatly reduce or eliminate processed foods from your diet if you want to obtain mental wellness. If you currently have more than four servings of sugar/starches in your diet each day, follow the chart below to minimize the withdrawal effect.

Program to Reduce Sugar/Starches Gradually	
Week 1	4 Servings/Day
Week 2	3 Servings/Day
Week 3	2 Servings/Day
Week 4	1 Serving/Day
Week 5	0 Servings/Day

Artificial Sweetener Addiction & Withdrawal

Aspartame is a neurotoxin, and directly impacts the brain. Aspartame has been linked to a host of physical and mental problems. Similar to sugar, artificial sweeteners such as aspartame and Splenda (sucralose), are addictive and can hinder mental health when suddenly removed from the diet. Although these artificial sweeteners are detrimental to both mental and physical health, you will want to gradually reduce them as well to minimize the overall withdrawal effect. Survey how much you currently have in your diet, and create a plan to gradually reduce these over the first four weeks, until you are no longer consuming artificial sweeteners. Artificial sweeteners are hidden in chewing gum, candies, cereals, yogurt, diet sodas, and many more foods.

Although artificial sweeteners, like aspartame and Splenda, are like poison to the body, they are addictive and can result in terrible withdrawal symptoms if removed suddenly. Keep this in mind and consider gradually reducing the amount of artificial sweeteners in your diet until you are no longer consuming them, and then keep them out. This is not something you will even want to have on occasion, as it is a chemical and toxic to the brain.

Review of Optimal Mental Health Nutrition Plan

Review of Basic Dietary Plan for Optimal Mental Health

BASIC DIETARY PLAN REVIEW

- ✓ Eat **3 meals** per day and **2 snacks**
- ✓ Meals should contain **20-25 grams of healthy protein**, unlimited healthy fats (depending on ability to digest them), and vegetables
- ✓ Snacks are fruit
- ✓ Additional protein and fat can be eaten 20 minutes following your snack if you are still hungry
- ✓ Occasional beans and/or rice can be included in your diet in small quantities
- ✓ Adequate **clean water** is important for mental health
- ✓ Supplements should be included to optimize mental health
  - ○ Fish Oil: **3-6 grams/day** taken throughout the day with meals
  - ○ Digestive Supplements: You will learn which digestive supplements are best for you in the section on digestive health.
- ✓ Guidelines to reducing gluten/casein/sugar/artificial sweeteners will be given in the following section. It's important to remove these from the diet gradually to minimize the withdrawal effect.

Remove Common Food Allergens that can have a negative effect on mental health

Here is a list of foods to remove from your diet in order to optimize mental health:

- Wheat/Gluten
- Milk/Casein (not butter unless lactose intolerant)
- Nuts
- Soy
- Corn
- Any other known food you have a sensitivity to

Gradually Reduce Gluten/Casein to Minimize Withdrawal Effect:

Program to Reduce Gluten/Casein Gradually	
Week 1	4 Servings/Day
Week 2	3 Servings/Day
Week 3	2 Servings/Day
Week 4	1 Serving/Day
Week 5	0 Servings/Day

Gradually Reduce Sugar/Starches to Minimize Withdrawal Effect:

Program to Reduce Sugar/Starches Gradually	
Week 1	4 Servings/Day
Week 2	3 Servings/Day
Week 3	2 Servings/Day
Week 4	1 Serving/Day
Week 5	0 Servings/Day

Gradually Reduce Aspartame/Splenda to Minimize Withdrawal Effect

Chapter 8

Optimal Mental Health Nutrition Plan
Breakdown of Food Choices and Meals

List of Allowed Foods

Protein: It is important that you choose meats that have come from animals that are fed a healthy diet, get exercise, and are not given hormones or antibiotics. It is best, whenever possible, to get meats from a local farm, where you can observe and learn their practices. Otherwise, choose meats/eggs that are labeled the following way:

- **Grass-fed organic beef**: You want beef from an animal that is able to wander the land and eat from it (cows are meant to eat grass, which increases the omega-3 content of the meat; this allows them to get exercise as well). Conventional meats contain antibiotics and hormones which you do not want. Antibiotics affect the health of your digestive tract (more about that in Phase Two), and hormones impact your hormone balance and can ultimately affect your brain chemistry. Cows that have been mostly grain-fed also contain a much higher ratio of inflammatory fats.

- **Pastured or Free-Range Organic Chicken/Eggs**: This means that the chickens have been allowed to roam the land, get exercise, and eat off the land, as opposed to being caged. Pastured chickens are typically not fed antibiotics. Look for meats that say 'no antibiotics given'. Caged chickens are often crammed in with other chickens and do not get exercise, and are often fed antibiotics because they are more apt to have problems due to their living situation. This affects the health of the egg as well as the meat of the chicken. This, in turn, impacts the health of your body. It is illegal to give chickens hormones, so those packages that promote no hormones given but do not say anything about antibiotics, are a marketing ploy. Look for free-range or pastured organic chicken/eggs that are not given antibiotics. Finding a local farm that raises their chickens with these practices is always preferred over the supermarket.

- **Bison/Buffalo**: Bison are not given hormones or antibiotics, and are typically given plenty of land to roam in. For this reason, bison/buffalo is a great option to choose. It tends to be quite a bit more expensive unfortunately. You would like to choose one that says grass-fed as oppose to grain. When an animal is grass-fed, the content of omega-3 fats increases greatly, compared to omega-6 fats. We need a proper balance of fats in our diets; however, the American diet has emphasized a great deal more omega-6 fats, which promote inflammation in the body, verses omega-3 fats that are anti-inflammatory. Therefore, it's important to get more omega-3 fats to compensate. Omega-3 fats are important for brain health.

- **Venison (Deer)**: This is best if you or a friend have actually hunted the meat yourself. I don't like the idea of getting this meat from a farm. The more in the wild, the better and fresher. An animal in the wild will naturally eat what it is meant to and what is good for it. This improves the quality of the meat greatly. If you have a friend or relative who is a hunter, this may be a great option for you if you like the taste of venison.

- **Lamb**: Choose lamb meat from animals that are able to eat off the land. Lambs are also not given hormones or antibiotics, so this is a great option to choose.

- **Free-Range Organic Turkey**: For the same reasons as mentioned above for chicken.

- **Wild Meats**: Great sources of protein for same reasons as mentioned regarding deer.

- **Organic Ham, Pork, and Bacon**: You want to eat the meat from pigs that have plenty of space to get exercise and are fed a healthy diet. When cooking pork, it is important to marinate the meat overnight in apple cider or balsamic vinegar in order to break it down. Studies have shown that pork when it was not marinated caused the blood to coagulate (stick together), leading to potential blocking of the vessels. However, when marinated this did not occur. Other meats were tested and they did not cause the blood to coagulate whether or not they were marinated.[1] Choose ham and bacon that is free of nitrates.

- **Wild-Caught Fish/Seafood**: It's important that you choose wild-caught fish instead of farm-raised. Wild-caught fish contains a much higher ratio of omega-3 fats, which are so important to the health of the brain, compared to farm-raised. Unfortunately, we cannot avoid all contaminants that are now in our oceans, due to pollution. As a result, it's important to choose a variety of proteins (from meats, eggs, and fish) throughout each week to get a variety of nutrients in your body in order to fuel your brain.

Healthy Fats: Choosing the proper fats is very important for your brain. Your brain is roughly 60% fat, mostly saturated fat. We've been brain-washed to believe that saturated fat is bad for us, but that is simply not true. The source of the fat is what is most important. Just because a fat is saturated does not mean it is bad. Coconut oil is one of the best fats you can cook with, and it is mostly saturated fat. Coconut oil has been shown to be anti-inflammatory, anti-fungal, anti-viral, anti-bacterial, and helps to boost the metabolism.[2] I recommend including coconut oil in your diet daily and cooking most things in it. Because it is saturated, it won't go bad when heated to high temperatures, which is a problem for other fats. Once you heat a polyunsaturated fat, it goes rancid. Polyunsaturated fats are very unstable and will go bad when exposed to light, heat, or oxygen. A rancid fat is damaging to the body. You want to avoid rancid fats. For that reason, vegetable oils are not recommended. This is difficult if you eat out at restaurants a lot, as most of the oils used in cooking your food are vegetable oils. Monounsaturated fats, such as olive oil, can tolerate low heat without going rancid; however, once they are heated to higher temperatures they are no longer good. Olive oil is great to sprinkle on after the food has been cooked or as a salad dressing. You can also add a saturated fat to olive oil when cooking, to protect the oil from going bad. Your brain needs the proper fats to function at its best, and this is a key component to your mental health. You will need to also avoid all hydrogenated, partially-hydrogenated, and trans-fats. Here is a list of the healthy fats you should be consuming regularly.

- **Virgin Organic Coconut Oil**: You want to choose an organic virgin coconut oil; it should taste and smell like coconuts. If you do not care for coconut, still give this a try as it is not overpowering in taste, and many who do not like coconut still love cooking in coconut oil.

- **Extra-Virgin Organic Olive Oil**: You want to choose a first-pressed, cold-pressed olive oil in a dark container. Olive oil will go bad when subjected to light, heat, and oxygen, so you want to purchase and keep this in a dark glass bottle, properly sealed. You can use this to cook in low temperatures only; however, adding a stable healthy saturated fat (such as coconut oil or organic butter) with the olive oil while cooking in slightly higher temperatures will help to keep the olive oil from going bad. Otherwise, this is great for salads. I often use olive oil, balsamic vinegar, sea salt, and garlic powder to dress my salads.

- **Organic Butter**: As long as you do not have a problem with lactose, you are free to use butter liberally, as long as it is organic. Butter is the fat part of milk from the cow. If you do not choose organic butter, then it is likely to contain some antibiotics, as cows are often given antibiotics to keep from getting infections from being over-milked and not allowed to get much exercise. Toxins are stored in fat tissues, and so the fat component (butter) of the milk is where many of the toxins will be. For this reason you want to choose organic. Organic (preferably raw) butter contains many nutrients and is a healthy source of fat.

- **Avocados**: Avocados are a great source of fat. They are great chopped up in a salad or as a side to a meal. I will often cut one up and add olive oil, balsamic vinegar, sea salt, and a little garlic powder or fresh garlic. If you are unfamiliar with avocados, choose ones that give just slightly when you squeeze them gently. If they are too mushy, they will likely be brown inside and you've just wasted your money. If they are hard as a rock, they are not close to being ripe yet. As with all produce, it's always best to get them locally (which depends on where you live) and picked closest to being ripe so that they contain the most amount of nutrients. That being said, even if that is not possible for you, avocados are still a great fat to eat.

- **Olives**: Choose organic.

- **Fat from healthy meat sources:** You will be getting fat in some of the meats that you choose and, as long as you chose healthy sources, then the fat from these meats is good for you.

- **Fat from fish/seafood:** As long as you have chosen healthy sources of seafood, then the fats that naturally occur with them are good for you. You will be supplementing with fish oil, as it is such a great source of omega-3 fats that are so vital to the health of the brain.

Produce: It is important to NOT eat any Genetically Modified foods. To determine whether your produce is genetically modified, you can look at the label. If it contains a five-digit number starting with an 8, then it is genetically modified. If it has a five-digit number starting with a 9, then it is organic. If it has a four-digit number starting with a 4, then it is conventionally grown with pesticides.

> 8: genetically-modified
> 9: organic
> 4: conventionally-grown with pesticides

To optimize success in this program, you want to choose organic whenever possible and totally avoid anything that is genetically-modified (GMO). Genetically-modified foods wreak havoc on the digestive tract, and will greatly hinder your ability to reach optimal mental health. For this reason, you need to avoid all genetically-modified foods. Finding a local organic farm near you is the best option for choosing your produce.

Vegetables: It is best to eat a variety of vegetables to obtain as many nutrients as possible. The requirement is a minimum of three servings per day. If you feel like having more, as long as you are not stuffing yourself go ahead. However, it is important that you do not put too much in your body at one time, as this will hinder your ability to digest the food. Here is a list of vegetables (it is not an exhaustive list). All vegetables are permitted on this program.

- Kale, spinach, all different lettuces, cabbage, sprouts, Brussels sprouts, fiddleheads
- Cucumber, broccoli, cauliflower, asparagus, fennel, peppers, onion, garlic, mushroom
- Starchy vegetables: all potatoes (including sweet), yams, squash, carrots, turnips, parsnips, peas, green beans, beets

Fruit: It is best to eat a variety of fruits. Local, organic, and in-season is always best, or you can choose organic frozen to optimize nutrient content. The requirement is a minimum of two servings of fruit eaten between meals as a snack. To optimize digestion, you do not want to eat fruit combined with your proteins and fat. Here is a list of fruits (it is not an exhaustive list). All fresh fruits are permitted on this program. Dried fruits are not recommended on this program, as many of them contain sulfites and have a high sugar content that can disrupt blood sugar balance.

- Blueberries, strawberries, raspberries, blackberries
- Apples, pears, grapes, banana
- Oranges, grapefruit, lemon, lime
- Peaches, nectarines, plums
- Pineapple, mango, papaya
- Kiwi, star fruit, pomegranate
- Watermelon, cantaloupe, muskmelon
- Tomato

Beans/Legumes: Some individuals may not do well consuming beans/legumes. This is something you will want to do a trial of to see how you handle these. All beans/legumes are allowed on this program, unless you determine you do not do well with them. Beans contain a lot of fiber, which may be problematic for some until you get your digestive system functioning properly (particularly the proper bacterial balance in the digestive tract, which will be addressed in Phase Two). It's best to purchase your beans and soak them, instead of purchasing canned. Canned foods often contain a plastic-derived liner that contains Bis-phenyl A, which is toxic to the body and can act as an endocrine disruptor, affecting your hormones. This is the reason you also do not want to drink water out of plastics or store your food in plastic.

Drinks: You will largely be consuming clean, filtered water throughout the day. Your goal is to drink half your body weight in fluid ounces each day, but not exceeding 100 fluid ounces. By drinking this amount of water, you will not likely want to drink much else. However, you may want something different from time to time, some of which can be included as part of your daily water intake:

- **Coconut Water:** This is a great source of electrolytes. Can be included as part of your daily water intake.
- **Coconut Milk:** Ideally not from a can. Unfortunately, many coconut milks are fortified with vitamin D2. Vitamin D2 can become toxic to the body; it's vitamin D3 that you want, not D2, so check the labels. Coconut milk is also great in soups and stir fry.
- **Hot Tea:** Be careful not to drink too much tea, as it contains fluoride; however, a glass of hot water with honey and cinnamon or honey with lemon and ginger is a great hot drink. You can also combine fresh ginger, turmeric, and honey for a great tasting drink. Warm lemon water is a great way to start the day, as it is a natural detoxifier. These hot drinks can be included as part of your daily water intake.

- **Hot Cocoa:** Made at home with cacao powder, coconut milk, honey/pure maple syrup, and gluten-free vanilla extract. Do not buy the packaged hot cocoa, as it contains many ingredients that are not optimal for mental health. This cannot be included as part of your daily water intake.

- **Organic Coffee**: Only in moderation if you must. Caffeine is known to produce anxiety and panic attacks, [3-7] so you will want to work to slowly decrease the caffeine in your diet if you ingest a lot. Caffeine also hinders the binding of GABA (the neurotransmitter responsible for helping you to relax) to receptor sites, thus hindering sleep.[8] Sleep-deprivation is detrimental to mental health and is one of the foundations for mental health. Decrease by a half a cup of coffee per week until you are no longer consuming coffee or drinking only one cup per day. Cannot be included as part of your daily water intake.

- **Fresh vegetables/fruit juices:** You don't want bottled juices from the market. Commercial juices often contain sugar and lack much nutrition, as the nutrient content goes down quickly after it is juiced. Fresh vegetables and/or fruit juices are good to consume if you are juicing the produce yourself. Fresh organic juice contains lots of nutrients that are easily absorbed into the digestive tract. Be sure to drink your juice soon after juicing it. It's ok to juice fruits and vegetables together as long as you are not also including fat and/or protein. You will need to be careful with throwing blood sugar levels off by drinking too much juice. Juicing removes the fiber, which is needed to help keep blood sugar stable. Making fruit or vegetable smoothies is a better option, as it keeps the fiber intact and helps to keep blood sugar stable.

- **Fruit smoothies:** This can be a great snack by including frozen and/or fresh fruit with water. Later on in the program you may be able to add things like yogurt, as it is a fermented protein, to these smoothies but not for now. Simply blend the fruit with water and a little bit of honey or maple syrup if desired. The water included in the smoothie can be counted as part of your daily water intake.

Other Foods Allowed:

Sweeteners: The following sweeteners are allowed in *moderation* in the program, but should not be combined with protein or fat. Use in fruit smoothies or add to tea.

- o Raw Honey: Great source of nutrients and very healing to the body.
- o Pure Maple Syrup: Contains multiple nutrients and is a great tasting sweetener.
- o Black Molasses: Great source of nutrients but has a strong taste.

Balsamic, Apple Cider, & Coconut Vinegar: Great for use in salad dressings and marinades.

Coconut Aminos: Use in place of soy sauce.

Coconut Flour: Can be used in place of white flour. Use for making gravy.

Herbs: All fresh and dried herbs are allowed.

Spices/Seasonings: Be sure to choose gluten-free versions. Use sea salt instead of refined white salt.

Homemade meat stock and bone broth: Made from meat and bones from a healthy meat source.

Gluten-Free Vanilla Extract: Can be used in making homemade hot cocoa.

Brown Rice: is allowed in moderation. Brown rice bread crumbs are great for making breaded chicken, fish, or pork. Limit brown rice to ½-cup servings no more than twice per week. If you have a lot of starches in your diet when you start this program, you can begin with more brown rice and gradually reduce the amount you eat each week to minimize any withdrawal or detox response.

Foods NOT PERMITTED on the Program:

This is not an exhaustive list. If you stick to the foods permitted on the program, then you should be ok. However, to simplify any questions you may have, here is a list of some foods not permitted.

- **Unhealthy fats:** Vegetable oils, hydrogenated fats, partially-hydrogenated fats, trans-fats, canola oil, soybean oil, fats from animals that have been given hormones and/or antibiotics, fats from farm-raised fish/seafood

- **Unhealthy protein sources** from animals that have been given hormones and/or antibiotics

- **Common food allergens:** Wheat/gluten, casein (milk, cheese, yogurt, ice cream), corn, nuts, and soy. Also keep out any food that you have a known allergy to that may not be on this list. Some of these things may be added back in to your diet at a later date, once the digestive system is functioning well, and as long as there is no sensitivity, such as raw, soaked nuts/seeds, raw milk (if tolerated), and organic corn.

- **Bread products:** Pasta, bread, crackers, cereal, oatmeal, etc.

- **Grains** are not allowed on the program except for rice.

- **Rice.** Brown rice bread crumbs for making certain breaded meals. Brown rice is allowed but limited to only two servings per week.

- **Sugar** or sugar-containing products.

- **Alcohol:** Causes an imbalance in blood sugar that can impact mood, as well as depletes much needed nutrients to the brain.

- **Bouillon cubes** (for making soup) often contain MSG and unwanted ingredients.

- **Soy sauce**

- **Commercial salad dressings & marinades:** Many contain bad fats and gluten. Make your own salad dressings and marinades.

Meal Ideas

Egg Meals

- **Omelet with mixed veggies** – Choose any vegetables and create an omelet cooked in coconut oil.

- **Eggs, bacon, and home fries** – Cook eggs any style you like in coconut oil or bacon grease. Dice up white or sweet potatoes and cook in coconut oil with sea salt.

- **Spinach Zucchini Egg Muffins** – Mix eggs, spinach, chopped zucchini, scallions, and fresh basil. Grease muffin pans well with butter and fill with mixture. Cook at 375 degrees for 15 minutes.

- **Steak & Eggs** – Great when you've just had steak the night before. Add some steak to an egg omelet with onions and peppers or any mixed vegetables. Cook in coconut oil.

Chicken Meals

- **Chicken Stir-Fry** – Cook any chicken (breast, thighs, or legs) and cut into small pieces. Cook assorted vegetables, like broccoli, mushrooms, onions, and garlic or red peppers, parsnips, sweet potato, and peas or sugar snap peas, carrots, onions, and peppers or any combination of vegetables that you like. Cook in coconut oil and add sea salt to taste.

- **Chicken Balls (kids love these)** – Using organic ground chicken, roll small balls in brown rice crumbs, garlic powder, sea salt, and oregano. Cook in coconut oil and/or butter and add more sea salt to taste. Serve with vegetables of any kind.

- **Grilled Chicken** – Season chicken with olive oil, organic butter, and multiple spices. Be sure to choose gluten-free spices. You can choose a chicken spice blend or use garlic powder, oregano, sea salt, and black pepper. Grill chicken until fully cooked. Eat with potato or any vegetable.

Ham/Pork/Bacon Meals

- **Ham Bone Lentil Soup** – Cook an organic gluten free ham. Save bone and some meat for soup. Rinse 1 (16 oz.) package of dried lentils. Place at the bottom of the crock pot. Next add the ham bone and 2 cups of diced ham, 1 cup sliced carrots, 1 cup chopped yellow onion, 2 ribs of celery, 2 cloves of garlic minced, 1 bay leaf, and ¼ cup chopped fresh parsley or 1 tsp dried parsley. Add water to cover (about 7 cups). Add sea salt and pepper to taste. Cook on high 4-5 hours or low 8-10 hours.

- **Pork Chops** – Marinate pork chops in apple cider or balsamic vinegar, olive oil, and gluten-free seasonings overnight. Grill until fully cooked. Eat with mixed greens/veggie salad.

- **Pork Roast** – Marinate pork roast overnight (as indicated in pork chops above). Place in crock pot with cut up onion, celery, carrots, and potatoes. Add 1-2 cups of water to keep moist. Cook on high 4-5 hours or low 8-10 hours until meat is tender.

Turkey Meals

- **Turkey Dinner with Coconut Flour Gravy** – Cook a full turkey and save bones for making soup later. Keep in freezer if you do not have time to make it soon. Broth made from the bones is very healthy. Eat turkey with coconut flour gravy. To make coconut flour gravy, slowly stir coconut flour into juices from the turkey on the stove top until it becomes thick to your liking. Eat with green beans, sweet potatoes, or other vegetables of your choice. Freeze excess turkey for use later.

- **Turkey Soup** – Place turkey bones in large pot on stove. Cover bones with water. Add 2 tbsp. of apple cider vinegar and sea salt. The vinegar helps to draw the minerals out of the bones. Add chopped onion, garlic, carrots, celery, or other vegetables to flavor. Cook on low for 24-48 hours. The longer it's cooked, the higher the mineral content of the broth. Once fully cooked, strain out bones and vegetables. Remove any meat and keep vegetables, but be careful to remove all the bones. Blend the remaining meat and vegetables in a blender and add back into soup. Add more chopped vegetables as you like, or simply save broth for making other soups later. Keep in refrigerator up to 4 days or freeze.

- **Turkey Salad** – Mix turkey (left over from turkey dinner) in a blender with olive oil, balsamic vinegar, and sea salt. Once blended add chopped celery. Serve on greens.

- **Ground Turkey Soup** – Cook ground turkey on the stove top in coconut oil. Add previously-made turkey broth or chicken broth. Add chopped green beans, sea salt, black pepper, garlic, and onions.

Beef Meals

- **Fiesta Chili** – Soak ½ a bag of black beans overnight in water then rinse. In a large pan heat 1 tbsp. of olive oil and a pat of butter. Add 1 chopped onion, 1 chopped green pepper, 1 chopped red pepper, 1 tsp. ground cumin, 1 tsp. minced garlic, 1 jar chipotle salsa, black beans, 2 diced tomatoes, 1 can (BPA-free) tomato paste plus 3 cans water, ½ tsp salt, and ½ tsp black pepper. Bring to a boil, reduce heat and simmer 30 minutes.

- **Tacos** – Cook ground beef until fully cooked. Add homemade seasoning (do not want to buy store bought unless you can find a healthy organic version) –include ground cumin, chili powder, garlic powder, paprika, cayenne pepper, sea salt, and ground pepper. Season ground beef and add a small amount of water. Using large lettuce leaves (like romaine) as a taco shell, fill with taco meat, sliced onions, tomatoes, and salsa.

- **Pot Roast** – Place pot roast in the crock pot and cover with salsa and chopped green peppers. Add 1-2 cups of water.

Cook on high for 4-5 hours or low for 8-10 hours. Can also cook this with chopped onions, carrots, and potatoes.

- **Beef Burgers** – Cook on grill or on stove top. I like to make mini flat burgers cooked in coconut oil on the stove top and flattened with a spatula. Add onions and mushrooms cooked in butter over top of the burgers. You can also cook ¼ lb. burgers on the grill. Add onion, tomato, and lettuce. Use large lettuce leaves as a bun.

- **Hamburger Vegetable Soup** – Cook 2 lbs. of ground beef and 2 cups of chopped onion. Add 2 cups of diced potatoes, 2 cups sliced carrots, 2 cups shredded cabbage, 6-8 cups water, 1 ½ - 2 ½ tbs. sea salt, ½ tsp. basil, ½ tsp. thyme, and 2 bay leaves. Bring to a boil. Reduce heat, cover and simmer for 2-4 hours. Check periodically and add more water if needed. Remove bay leaves and serve.

Bison/Buffalo Meals

- **Bison Burgers** – cook the same as a beef burger
- **Bison Tacos** – cook same as beef tacos

Lamb Meals

- **Leg of Lamb**
- **Ground lamb with kale** – Cook chopped onion and kale in coconut oil. Cook until the kale becomes limp. In a separate pan, cook ground lamb and fold in chopped garlic. Once fully cooked, add to the kale and onion.

Venison Meals

- **Venison Stir-Fry** – Slice venison flank and cook on stove top in coconut oil. Cut into strips. Cook sliced onions and mixed peppers, and add to the flank.

Wild-Caught Fish/Seafood Meals

- **Sashimi** (from a fresh wild-caught source) – my favorites are salmon, scallops, and tuna. Squeeze the juice of lemon over and dip in coconut aminos instead of soy sauce.

- **Breaded Cod or Haddock** – Dip fish in egg then in brown rice crumbs with seasonings. Cook in coconut oil. Enjoy vegetables or a salad with your fish.

- **Scallops & Brussels Sprouts** – Cook bacon in large skillet. Once cooked remove bacon but keep bacon fat in pan. Cook Brussels sprouts until tender. Add back in the bacon chopped. In separate pan, cook scallops on each side being careful not to overcook. Add to the Brussels sprouts and enjoy!

Snack Ideas: On this program, your snack is a fruit of your choice. However, you can also opt to make a fruit smoothie for your snack. Here are some fruit smoothie ideas:

In a blender mix the following ingredients:

Berry Bliss Smoothie
Mixed Frozen Organic Berries
Banana
Water

Tropical Smoothie
Fresh Mango
Fresh Pineapple
Ice
Water

Shopping List

This list is also included at the end of the book for quick reference.

Healthy Protein Sources:
- ✓ Grass-Fed Organic Beef
- ✓ Pastured or Free-Range Organic Eggs/Chicken
- ✓ Bison/Buffalo
- ✓ Venison/Deer
- ✓ Lamb
- ✓ Wild Meats
- ✓ Free-Range Organic Turkey
- ✓ Organic Nitrate-Free Ham, Pork, & Bacon
- ✓ Wild-Caught Fish/Seafood

Healthy Fat Sources:
- ✓ Organic Virgin Coconut Oil
- ✓ Extra-Virgin Organic Olive Oil
- ✓ Organic Butter
- ✓ Organic Olives
- ✓ Avocados
- ✓ Healthy Fats from Healthy Meats

Vegetables: All are permitted. Choose organic, local, in-season or organic frozen. Corn is a grain and is not permitted.

Fruits: All are permitted. Choose organic, local, in-season or organic frozen.

Beans: All beans are permitted. Choose dry beans and soak instead of canned.

Drinks:
- ✓ Coconut Water
- ✓ Coconut Milk
- ✓ Organic Coffee (in moderation)

Other Allowed Items:
- ✓ Raw Honey
- ✓ Pure Maple Syrup
- ✓ Black Molasses
- ✓ Balsamic, Apple-Cider, or Coconut Vinegar
- ✓ Coconut Aminos
- ✓ Coconut Flour
- ✓ Gluten-Free Spices/Seasonings
- ✓ Sea Salt
- ✓ Gluten-Free Vanilla Extract
- ✓ Raw Cacao or Cocoa Powder
- ✓ Herbs & Sprouts
- ✓ Brown Rice Bread Crumbs

Journaling: Keeping a food/mood log is very important to monitoring your progress, particularly with mental health issues. It's human nature, at times, to have a bad day and think that all is lost (especially if your brain chemistry is less than optimal), but if you look back at your journal you may just find the key to your bad day, as well as remind yourself that you've been doing a whole lot better since you first started. This will give you the motivation you need to continue instead of throwing in the towel. I have included a food journal page to be copied and used to record your daily food intake or you can purchase the Optimal Mental Health Nutrition Plan Food Journal separately. They are designed to help remind you of what you need to eat each meal and snack, as well as remind you to take your supplements. You will also keep track of your mood throughout the day. This will serve as a great way to keep track of your progress.

Record your mood throughout the day as indicated with things such as good, happy, sad, anxious, depressed, irritable, excited, etc. Feed your mind positive thoughts and include activities daily that help relieve stress and bring joy into your life. At the end of each day, record three good things that happened to you that day. This is a simple exercise that could have profound benefits by keeping your brain focused on the positive aspects of your life, which naturally benefits brain chemistry.

Food/Mood Log (make copies of this page or use the Optimal Mental Health Nutrition Plan Food Journal sold separately)

Day _____ Date _____

Breakfast: Protein _____ Fat _____
Vegetable _____
Supplements (check off): ☐ Fish Oil (1-2 grams with meal)
                              ☐ Digestive Supplements (with meal)
Mood: _____

Snack: Fruit _____ Other _____

Lunch: Protein _____ Fat _____
Vegetable _____
Supplements (check off): ☐ Fish Oil (1-2 grams with meal)
                              ☐ Digestive Supplements (with meal)
Mood: _____

Snack: Fruit _____ Other _____

Dinner: Protein _____ Fat _____
Vegetable _____
Supplements (check off): ☐ Fish Oil (1-2 grams with meal)
                              ☐ Digestive Aide (with meal)
Mood: _____

List three positive things that happened today:

1. _____
2. _____
3. _____

Never Give Up! With God ALL Things Are Possible!

Chapter 9

Optimal Mental Health Nutrition Plan
Phase One – Step 2: Digestive Health

MY STORY:

I was chronically constipated as a child, having one bowel movement every two weeks. Growing up, I did not know this was not normal. I would describe my bowel movements as hard, rabbit-like pellets. I would also have a very short window of opportunity to eliminate. If I did not get to the bathroom within that short window, the urge would pass and who knows when it would come again. My stomach would make terrible growling noises, not when I was hungry, but always after I ate. When I was in my early 20s, I noticed that my stomach would bloat all the time. I would eat something and feel like I was pregnant, and could visibly see my stomach distended. I became sensitive to more and more foods, and was unable to eat out without bloating and being in pain. I also experienced extreme fatigue as a result, and emotional distress. I was unable to eat many foods and so I did not eat out for four years. I eliminated all bread from my diet until I realized that it was the gluten in the foods that was causing a lot of trouble for me and discovered that gluten is hidden in many foods. I also eliminated milk, cheese, corn, soy, and nuts. Eliminating these foods helped to reduce my symptoms greatly and helped me to feel better physically and mentally however, it did not completely eliminate my mental health problems. I discovered that I had a severe HCL (hydrochloric acid) deficiency and learned the things I needed to do to heal my digestive system. Eliminating gluten and casein had a tremendous impact on my mental health and also helped to eliminate nightmares that I'd had since I was a child. Restoring my digestive system greatly impacted my well-being and resulted in an improvement in my bowel movements from once every two weeks to two to three times per day.

Health of your Digestive Tract

Let's begin by discussing the nutritional foundation, digestive health, in order to get a better understanding of why this is so important to your success.

Determining Digestive Problems

Eating a healthy diet to nourish your brain and body is only half the battle. Your digestive tract is responsible for the other half. This is where foods are broken down into nutrients, and then absorbed into the blood stream and ushered throughout the body where needed, including the brain. Our brains need to be well nourished in order to function properly for overall mental well-being. You will determine the health of your digestive system based on a test you can do at home as well as symptom check lists. This will give you a good indication of where you are starting from and then you will learn what you can do to optimize digestion.

The Beet Test (to determine transit time)

Transit time is the amount of time it takes for food to go through your entire digestive system and exit the body from the time it enters your mouth. Optimal transit time is between 19 and 24 hours. That means what you eat should be fully digested, nutrients absorbed, and waste products eliminated 19-24 hours after you eat it. If things are moving too quickly or too slowly through the body that is a problem. You can determine your transit time by doing The Beet Test in the privacy of your home. You will need to purchase two medium to large fresh red/purple beets. Some of you may not like the taste of beets but if you can manage it just this one time they do not have to be a regular part of your dietary plan unless you like beets. I do recommend including them in your diet, as they have many health benefits. If you have an allergy to beets then DO NOT use this test. You can use other foods to measure transit time, such as a green drink, but beets are much easier to see when they come out the other end. Once you have your beets, you can eat them in any of the following ways: raw, pan fried (in good oils), baked, or steamed but not boiled. You need the red color to stay intact. Eat the beets (all of them) with your meal and record the date and time that you eat them in the chart below:

	Date	Time
Beets Eaten	_____	_____
First see red in stool	_____	_____
Last see red in stool	_____	_____
Transit Time:	_____	

Consuming this amount of beets will produce a red stool. Watch your stool. Record when you first see red. Please do not be alarmed; you are not bleeding. Continue to watch your stool and record the last time you see red in your stool. The difference between when you first ate the beets until the last time you see red in your stool is your total transit time. Even if you see red in multiple stools it is the last time you see the red that gives you the total transit time.

This gives you a starting point for digestion. So what happens if transit time is not optimal?

< 19 hours: This means that things are moving too quickly through your digestive system. When food moves too quickly through your digestive tract it hinders nutrient absorption. This typically occurs because digestion is not functioning properly to break down the food. This results in the food becoming toxic in the gut. When this occurs the best thing the body can do is get the toxic waste out as soon as possible with diarrhea. The quicker the food goes through the body the greater the problem.

>24 hours: This means that food is staying in your digestive tract too long resulting in toxins being produced and absorbed into the body.

Both of these situations need to be addressed and have a similar starting point. If these recommendations do not resolve the situation and result in an optimal transit time, more action needs to be taken and may involve other dietary changes (such as identifying other food allergens), and/or adjusting supplementation, until the digestive system is functioning properly. This may take some time. If you are having difficulty obtaining an optimal transit time while following the program, it is recommended to see a qualified Nutritional Practitioner to assist you in personalizing your program for you, and to identify any other underlying root issues. Go to **www.GetAtTheRoots.com** or **www.NutritionalTherapy.com** to find a Nutritional Practitioner to assist you.

Even if you have a perfect transit time you will still need to work on optimizing your digestion in order to obtain nutrients to feed your brain. Please follow the guidelines provided towards the end of this chapter to optimize digestion.

Why You Need Stomach Acid

The stomach is the most acidic organ in the body for a reason. Our stomachs need to be acidic so that they can properly break down the food that we consume. Problems arise when our stomach is not acidic enough. More often than not acid reflux or heartburn is due to a lack of acid instead of too much. Stomach pain, bloating, constipation, and diarrhea are also problems that can arise due to a lack of stomach acid. Let me explain. Our brain signals our body to produce hydrochloric acid in the stomach when we are in a relaxed state. When we eat, we should be sitting down and relaxing, and allowing the body to produce the proper amounts of acid and enzymes, in order to digest our food. However, many people run in to trouble because they are eating on the go or eating while they work. This disrupts our body's ability to properly produce the acid and enzymes needed.

What happens if we do not have the proper acid in the stomach and subsequent enzymes in the small intestine to break down our food? Food stays in the stomach too long and doesn't get broken down properly and causes damage. When there is not enough acid in the stomach then it sits in the stomach too long. The body does not want to release it to the small intestine until it's properly broken down. Have you ever had that feeling when your stomach felt like a rock and the food was just sitting in there not digesting? Well, as the food sits there, the carbohydrates start to ferment, proteins begin to putrefy, and fats become rancid. The end result is toxic waste in your gut. The gases produced as this occurs may press up against the upper esophageal sphincter resulting in acid rising up into your esophagus causing you pain or better known as heart burn. The esophagus is not meant to be acidic and even though the stomach is not acidic enough to digest the food properly at that time it is still far more acidic than the esophagus. The best thing that the body could do at this point is release the toxic waste from the body as quickly as possible with diarrhea. Our body naturally wants to get the toxic waste out of the body as soon as possible so that it causes the least amount of damage. When this happens the body is unable to obtain nutrients from the food eaten, and likely damage was done to the lining of the digestive tract. It doesn't always result in heartburn and/or diarrhea. I've known plenty of individuals, including myself, who did not produce the proper amount of acid in their stomach and the damage in the digestive tract resulted in the opposite problem of constipation. Either way if you are experiencing symptoms of digestive distress (stomach pain, heart burn, bloating, constipation, and/or diarrhea) you have a problem. These are all signs that something is going wrong. It is important to work on optimizing digestion if you want to optimize mental health because this is where nutrients come in to supply your brain.

Determining Gallbladder Function

This is a critical component to overall digestive health and to mental well-being as the gallbladder is responsible for holding bile which is needed to break down fat. Healthy fats are vital to the health of the body and the brain. They are needed to manufacture brain chemistry and hormones. Getting adequate healthy fat in the diet is only half the solution. The other half is being able to break them down so that you are able to obtain the benefits from them. When the gallbladder has been removed or is not functioning properly important steps need to be taken to compensate for the inability to properly digest fats. Let me begin by explaining how the gallbladder functions. The liver makes bile and sends it to the gallbladder to be stored. Each time that you eat fat, the gallbladder contracts to release bile into the small intestine in order to break down the fats in the food consumed. This is good and important. Whoever said that the gallbladder is not needed is not correct. You can survive without one but digestion is hindered and it ultimately affects the health of the body and potentially the brain. God put a gallbladder in our bodies for a reason. If you have had yours removed don't lose heart there are things you can and need to do in order to obtain optimal mental health.

Gallbladder Removed: If you have had your gallbladder removed it is important to assist your body in breaking down fats. The liver still creates bile however; you no longer have a storage area to keep it in to be released when the time is needed. As a result, the bile released by the liver is not adequate to properly digest all the fats consumed in your meal. The gallbladder would normally contract based on the amount of fat in the meal however, the liver is unable to do that so there is just a small drip of bile being released into the small intestine. This is not enough to properly digest your fats. Those who do not have a gallbladder often do well to supplement with bile in order to assist the body in breaking down fats. I typically recommend a supplement that contains ox bile. *I would not attempt to consume the fats in this program that are so necessary for mental health without this supplement if you do not have a gallbladder. Doing so will result in mal-digestion of fat and further damage in the digestive tract and likely discomfort and diarrhea or digestive distress.*

Gallbladder Dysfunction: How do you know if you have a gallbladder that is not functioning optimally? Consider the checklist of symptoms below to indicate whether or not you may have a gallbladder that is not properly functioning. When the gallbladder is functioning properly the bile is thin and is easily released from the gallbladder when it contracts every time fat is eaten. If an individual has gone on a low or no fat diet for a period of time the bile can become thick and viscous. When this happens it is difficult to get the proper amount of bile out of the gallbladder making it difficult to digest the fat in the meal as well as potentially causing stones to develop.

Symptoms of Gallbladder Dysfunction (check all that apply):
- ☐ Stomach upset by greasy foods
- ☐ Headaches over the eyes
- ☐ Nausea, motion sickness
- ☐ History of morning sickness
- ☐ Light or clay-colored stool
- ☐ Greasy or shiny stools
- ☐ Pain between shoulder blades
- ☐ Gallbladder attacks (pain/tightening under right rib cage)
- ☐ Bitter taste in mouth after meals

If you are experiencing gallbladder dysfunction it is important that you consume healthy fats in moderation (still three times per day but smaller quantities) to begin with as you work to restore the health of the gallbladder. Taking a supplement to help thin the bile (such as Biotics Beta-TCP) can be helpful. Beets, apples, and ginger are also helpful to keeping the gallbladder functioning properly. Including these in the diet on a regular basis, along with healthy fats, will help to keep the gallbladder healthy.

Guidelines to Optimize Digestive Health

1. **Relax and eat slowly.** This helps the body to be able to produce the proper stomach acid and enzymes needed to break down your food.
2. **Chew food well.** The more you chew your food, the less your body has to do to break it down. Assist your body and optimize nutrient absorption by chewing your food well.
3. **Drink adequate water to hydrate the body.** If things are moving too quickly you will be more apt to become dehydrated. On the other hand, if things are moving too slowly

it may be due to dehydration. Stay hydrated to optimize digestion.

4. **You will be adding fermented foods in Phase Two in order to optimize digestion**. It's important to not start them now unless you have them in your diet regularly already as this can cause a detox reaction that can hinder your state of mind. You will want to do things gradually for optimal success.

5. **Removing the common food allergens**. This will help tremendously in the health of the digestive system and correcting a less than optimal transit time. You also want to identify any other foods that are problematic for you, and remove them from your diet, while working to heal the digestive tract.

6. **Eat fruit alone**. Fruit digests quickly. Proteins and fats take a lot longer to digest. For this reason you do not want to combine them. It's okay to add a small amount of honey or pure maple syrup to those smoothies as they digest rather quickly as well. Combining fruit with protein or fat can hinder your body's ability to digest properly and hinder your progress.

Supplement Recommendations: The success of the program is greatly enhanced by the addition of supplements to aid digestion and optimize nutrition to the brain. You can opt to find/use supplements of your choice; however, all supplements are not created equal. I recommend using high-quality nutritional supplements. The products below are a professional line of supplements and you will need to consult with a Nutritional Practitioner to personalize a program for you. These are the products I recommend based on their quality. Your Nutritional Practitioner may recommend similar products that would work best for you. Here is an example of what your program may look like:

General (for those who have their gallbladder and are not portraying symptoms of gallbladder dysfunction)	
Supplement Name	**Recommended Dose**
Biotics Betaine Plus HP and/or Biotics Hydrozyme	1-3 per meal *
Biotics Biomega-3 (fish oil)	3-6 per day with meals

No Gallbladder (for those who have had their gallbladder removed)	
Supplement Name	**Recommended Dose**
Biotics Betaine Plus HP and/or Biotics Hydrozyme	1-3 per meal *
Biotics Biomega-3	3-6 per day with meals
Biotics Beta-Plus	1-2 per meal

Gallbladder Dysfunction (for those who are experiencing symptoms of gallbladder dysfunction)	
Supplement Name	**Recommended Dose**
Biotics Betaine Plus HP and/or Biotics Hydrozyme	1-3 per meal *
Biotics Biomega-3	3-6 per day with meals
Biotics Beta-TCP	1-2 per meal

*Or more based on recommendations by a qualified Nutritional Practitioner

Supplements to Aid Digestion:

- **Hydrochloric Acid and Enzymes:** Most individuals will benefit from adding a supplement that includes these items. (Biotics Betaine Plus HP, Biotics Hydrozyme)

- **Ox Bile** (Biotics Beta-Plus): Can be very helpful if an individual has had their gallbladder removed.

- **Supplement for Gallbladder Dysfunction**: Biotics Beta-TCP contains beet powder to help thin the bile and restore it to its proper functioning. You can also consume beets, apples, and ginger on a regular basis in order to help bring the gallbladder back to proper functioning.

To have a personalized supplement program designed for you by a qualified Nutritional Professional contact **www.GetAtTheRoots.com.**

Chapter 10

Optimal Mental Health Nutrition Plan
Phase One – Step 3: Hydration

Water is so important to the health of our bodies. Our bodies are 50-70% water. We need water to usher nutrients throughout the body and brain. Without adequate hydration our brains may not be getting properly nourished through the foods we eat. Water also helps to eliminate toxins from the body and toxicity in the body can negatively impact mental health. The first signs of dehydration are typically fatigue and potentially headaches. However, dehydration can also lead to anxiety, depression, and mood changes among many other health problems.

Multiple studies have shown that dehydration can have a negative impact on mood with as low as a 1.3% reduction in hydration levels.[1-5] We typically don't feel thirsty until we have a water loss of 1-2% from our bodies. Many people also often mistake thirst for hunger and may reach for sugar or unhealthy foods when their body is really thirsty. Keeping the body hydrated will help to keep you from reaching for those foods that will deplete your body of nutrients and have a negative effect on mental health.

To ensure adequate water intake follow the guidelines below:

Your goal is to work up to drinking half of your body weight in fluid ounces each day up to but not exceeding 100 fl. oz. You want to increase this gradually so as to not overtax the kidneys. Slowly increase your current water intake by four ounces each day until you reach your goal.

To determine your daily water needs use the formula below:

Your weight _____ / 2 = _____ fluid ounces daily

Start each day with at least one to two glasses of water before eating breakfast. Then disperse the remainder of your water intake for the day throughout the day. It is best to drink between and before meals. If you drink water during your meal you can hinder optimal digestion by diluting the gastric juices.

Here are some guidelines to follow when planning your water intake for the day:

1. Drink 10 ounces of water upon awakening. Drinking warm lemon water at this time is a great way to begin cleansing the body first thing in the morning.

2. Then take the amount that you need to drink for the remainder of the day and divide it by four. You should strive to consume this amount of water the hour before each meal/snack based on the five total meals and snacks per day (not including breakfast as you have already had 10 ounces of water upon awakening). Review the chart on the following page to see examples of how this works out for the day.

3. When you are exercising, depending on the intensity, you will need to add in more water on top of your daily requirement.

4. Sip water with meals as drinking a lot of water with your meal will dilute the digestive juices and may hinder overall digestion.

5. Always listen to your body. Thirst is a sign that you are dehydrated. Many of us do not recognize the thirst signal and often think we are hungry.

6. Water should be ingested throughout the day.

Recommended Water Intake Chart

	Daily Water Requirement (in fluid ounces)					
	50	60	70	80	90	100
Upon Awakening Before Breakfast	10	10	10	10	10	10
The Hour Before Snack 1	10	12	15	17	20	22
The Hour Before Meal 2	10	12	15	17	20	22
The Hour Before Snack 2	10	12	15	17	20	22
The Hour Before Meal 3	10	12	15	17	20	22

It is also very important that you drink clean, filtered water out of glass or stainless steel and not from plastic as it can leach chemicals into the water. This is important as you do not want to be creating more damage with the water that you are drinking by drinking unfiltered water that may contain bacteria, chemicals, and chlorine.

It is extremely important to hydrate the body so that hormones and nutrients can be delivered as well as toxins can be removed. Making sure that you are getting adequately hydrated each day is a simple step you can take to optimize mental health.

Be Careful of Dehydrating Beverages

Beverages that contain caffeine such as coffee and tea along with prepackaged fruit juices are dehydrating. For this reason you will want to minimize or eliminate the use of these beverages in your diet.

Chapter 11

Optimal Mental Health Nutrition Plan
Phase Two (4+Weeks)
Your Microbiome & Sleep

Step 1: Your Microbiome

"Your gut literally serves as your second brain, and even produces more of the neurotransmitter serotonin—known to have a beneficial influence on your mood—than your brain does, so maintaining a healthy gut will benefit your mind as well as your body." Dr. Mercola [1]

In this phase, you will be introducing foods to heal the gut lining and restore bacterial balance to the body. This is a key component to the overall health of your body and mind. The gut produces approximately 80-90% of the body's serotonin; our natural mood stabilizer.[2] Low serotonin has been associated with depression.[3] Because of this, it is essential to consider the health of the digestive tract when seeking to obtain mental wellness. You may have heard it said the gut is the body's second brain. This term was coined by Dr. Michael Gershon, a researcher in the field of neurogastroenterology, who has studied the gut-brain connection and is author of the book, *The Second Brain*.[4] The second brain is a mass of neural tissue in the gut also known as the enteric nervous system. Much like the central nervous system, which sends messages from the brain via the spinal cord throughout the body and back, the enteric nervous system is a sheath of neurons that runs from the esophagus to the anus containing far more neurons than the peripheral or nervous system.[5] The gut (enteric nervous system) relays messages to the central nervous system via the vagus nerve to the brain. Therefore if the digestive system is not functioning properly it signals the brain and we often don't feel well mentally which we sometimes refer to as a "nervous stomach". If the digestive tract is unable to properly digest foods this can lead to toxin production as well as bacterial imbalances resulting in toxicity in both the gut and the brain impacting mental health. Considering the health of your digestive system is therefore vital in the process of reaching optimal mental wellness.

There have been many studies done on intestinal permeability, bacteria, and the gut-brain connection to depression and anxiety. Studies have shown that those with depression may have a compromised intestinal barrier.[6-7] The permeability of the intestinal wall is increased with psychological stress and excessive exercise.[8-10] Several studies have been done on intestinal bacteria and the brain. One study found that after 30 days of consuming probiotic bacteria the result was a decrease in anxiety and depression.[11] Many other studies have also shown a connection between beneficial bacteria and a reduction in depression and anxiety.[12-14]

There are two types of intestinal bacteria that produce the neurotransmitter GABA which is our natural relaxer.[15] Both GABA and serotonin help us to maintain stable mental health as GABA helps us to relax and serotonin is important for our feelings of well-being. This may give us insight into the possibility of minimizing anxiety and depression by restoring the integrity of the intestinal wall and restoring healthy bacterial balance. I've personally witnessed clients who, after going on high doses of antibiotics, suffered mental health problems including anxiety and depression and would say they just don't feel like themselves anymore. Antibiotics destroy both the good and bad bacteria and can result in bacterial imbalances in the digestive tract. Restoring a healthy microbiome is necessary to restoring one to optimal mental and physical health.

In order to create a healthy microbiome in your digestive tract you will be introducing homemade bone broths and fermented foods. It is important to your overall progress to introduce these foods slowly to minimize the detoxification and/or healing reaction.

Bone Broth to Heal the Digestive Tract Lining & Nourish the Body

Bone broth is becoming increasingly more popular as it has many health benefits. Homemade bone broth contains minerals and gelatin both of which are very healing to the body and particularly the digestive tract. You will want to introduce bone broth into your diet according to the chart below:

How to Introduce Bone Broth
Week 1 of Phase Two: Begin with ½ cup of bone broth per day every other day for the first week.
Week 2: If you are feeling good with this increase to ½ cup per day for this week.
Week 3: Alternate 1 cup and ½ cup per day.
Week 4: Increase to 1 cup per day.

Beyond week four you will want to continue to include a minimum of one cup of bone broth per day. You can add the broth to soups or drink alone.

To make bone broth: Take the bones of a grass-fed cow (for beef broth) or a pastured organic chicken or turkey and place them in a large pot. Cover with clean, filtered water. Add one to two tablespoons of apple cider vinegar and sea salt (you can add more sea salt later to taste). Bring to a boil then cook on low for 24-48 hours. Remove bones and save broth. You can freeze some of the broth to be used later. You can also add chopped vegetables to this to add more flavor and nutrients when making your broth.

Fermented Foods to Restore Bacterial Balance

It is important to also introduce fermented foods very slowly to minimize detox reactions. You will not be consuming fermented dairy at this point in the program. You may be able to introduce it later depending on sensitivities.

How to Introduce Fermented Foods
Week 1 of Phase Two: Begin with 1 tbsp. of a cultured vegetable or 1 ounce of a fermented healthy drink (non-alcoholic).
Week 2: If you are feeling good, increase to 1 tbsp. twice per day or 1 ounce of a fermented drink twice per day. If you are not feeling well then decrease to ½ tbsp. per day and slowly increase each week by ½ tbsp.
Week 3: Increase to 1 tbsp. with each meal (three times per day) or 1 ounce of a fermented drink with each meal.
Week 4: Continue to consume 1 tbsp. with each meal or 1 ounce of a fermented drink with each meal. You may do well to increase this amount over time as your bacterial balance is restored to optimal health.

Introducing fermented foods too quickly particularly when there is a bacterial imbalance in the body may result in a detox reaction. This can have a negative impact on mental health as detox symptoms can include anxiety, irritability, fatigue, headaches, digestive symptoms, and other potential symptoms. For this reason you will want to gradually introduce them in order to minimize the detox response and maximize your chances of success in obtaining optimal mental health.

Fermented Food Options:

Any fermented vegetables or fermented Kombucha tea are options to include in your diet in order to build a healthy microbiome. Some examples are fermented sauerkraut, fermented pickles, fermented beets, fermented carrots, and fermented mixed vegetables. For drinks you can consume fermented teas, Beet Kvaas (fermented beet juice), fermented pickle juice, and others. Be sure to avoid fermented dairy at this point.

I learned a great deal about the benefits of cultured foods by going through the Certified Healing Foods Specialist (CHFS) Course with Nutritional Therapy Practitioner, Caroline Barringer. In December of 2012, she was interviewed by Dr. Mercola about the many benefits of these foods and in her interview made this recommendation,

> *"Just one quarter to one half cup of fermented veggies, eaten with one to three meals per day, can have a dramatically beneficial impact on your health."* [1] *Caroline Barringer, NTP*

This is a great recommendation to work up to over time particularly if you are not currently consuming fermented foods. I do not recommend starting here but follow the chart to gradually introduce fermented foods to minimize a detox reaction. Also in this interview Caroline gives great information on how to make your own cultured vegetables at home and discusses the many health benefits. Several years ago she teamed up with Nutritional Therapy Practitioner, Jennifer Pecot to start Immunitrition, a company that provides tasty cultured vegetables chock full of beneficial bacteria. [1,16]

I have also had the opportunity to go through the GAPS™ (Gut & Psychology Syndrome) Training with Dr. Natasha Campbell McBride. Dr. Campbell McBride worked as a neurologist and neurosurgeon for several years before she became a mother. It was at this point that she decided to go back to school for Nutrition when her child was diagnosed with autism at the age of three and the medical establishment told her that nothing could be done. Her studies led her to uncover the importance of a healthy gut to a healthy brain. She successfully helped her child lead a normal life free of autism and has continued on to help hundreds of children with autism and other mental health disorders by healing the digestive tract and restoring a healthy gut microbiome. She is a firm believer that a digestive system that does not have a healthy bacterial balance is causing toxicity in the body that ultimately leads to a toxic brain that is unable to function properly. Dr. Campbell-McBride has trained hundreds of GAPS™ Practitioners in multiple countries including the United States that help others to restore their mental health through the restoration of the digestive system. [17]

Phase Two: Step One Review (4 Weeks)

	Bone Broth	Fermented Foods
Week 1	Drink ½ cup every other day	1 tbsp. cultured vegetable or 1 oz. fermented drink daily
Week 2	Drink ½ cup every day	1 tbsp. cultured vegetable or 1 oz. fermented drink 2x per day
Week 3	Alternate 1 cup/ ½ cup daily	1 tbsp. cultured vegetable or 1 oz. fermented drink 3 x per day
Week 4	Drink 1 cup daily	Continue at 1 tbsp. or 1 oz. 3 x per day

Step 2: Optimizing Sleep

MY STORY: *Prior to figuring out my food sensitivities, stabilizing my blood sugar, and dealing with the toxins in my body, I had terrible sleep problems. I tried many things to get rest, but often found myself waking up after a few hours of sleep, unable to get back to sleep. My blood sugar would drop, causing me to wake up many nights. I would get up and eat something to help stabilize my blood sugar. I would then have a hard time getting back to sleep. Some nights, I barely slept at all. Once I started to eat to maintain blood sugar and remove food allergens, my sleep improved greatly. I also had terrible nightmares, which went away after eliminating food allergens and detoxing. Lack of sleep was definitely impacting my mental health. Resolving blood sugar, food allergies, improving the health of my liver, and reducing my toxin load has resulted in my body's ability to get a good night's rest.*

Evaluating Sleep

Ask yourself the following questions in order to evaluate your current sleep health:

- ☐ Do you get a minimum of eight hours of sleep per night?
- ☐ Do you wake up feeling rested?
- ☐ Do you sleep through the night without waking?
- ☐ Do you easily fall to sleep?

If you answered **YES** to all the above questions then consider yourself blessed and in a good position to create a stable foundation for mental health. If you answered **NO** to any or all of the questions above, then there are things you can do in order to optimize your mental health. You will want to determine what root issues may be hindering your ability to sleep, and work on improving them through the steps laid out here.

Many people with depression have difficulty sleeping. In fact, one of the symptoms of depression is insomnia. Many individuals with psychiatric illnesses have difficulty sleeping and a lack of sleep can lead to depression. These can be intertwined so it is important to address difficulties with sleep.

The purpose of sleep is for restoration of the body and brain. When you are unable to get adequate sleep then your body and brain suffer. There are multiple reasons that an individual may not be sleeping well. In this section I will address the things that pertain to nutrition as well as emotional health and give suggestions to help improve sleep. Sleep can be disrupted as a result of numerous things including blood sugar instability, toxicity, digestive problems, food sensitivities, imbalanced minerals, and stress. By working to build a healthy body and mind nutritionally you will be helping to improve your body's ability to sleep in order to restore health.

Blood Sugar Instability

If your blood sugar drops during sleep you may wake up. By eating a healthy balanced meal/snack prior to bed you can help your blood sugar to stay stable throughout the night. This program is designed to help you maintain blood sugar stability and should help those who have difficulty staying asleep as a result of their blood sugar dropping during the night. For those individuals who are waking due to low blood sugar, you should have a healthy balanced snack when you awaken to bring blood sugar levels back to normal. You will want to work on laying a good foundation of health and may need to work on bringing health to the adrenals in order to get long term benefits to keeping blood sugar stable. Adrenal health is addressed in the next phase of the program.

Toxicity

When we sleep our digestive systems relax and our bodies work to restore and also deal with toxins in the process. Individuals who are overloaded with toxins can then be awakened in the night if the body is overly burdened. Nightmares are also a potential sign of toxicity in the body. While I worked to heal, my overly toxic body was the last thing to finally be addressed. I knew that I was toxic, as I felt it, but all methods of detoxification left me feeling worse and so I aborted every detox program I started. I eventually discovered that this was due to my extremely sluggish digestive system. As a result, when I would attempt a detox program and the toxins were being pulled from my tissues to be eliminated from the body, my body was becoming more toxic as it was unable to eliminate them through the digestive tract. The skin is also a major eliminating organ and I learned that my acne was a result of both food sensitivities and the toxins moving out of my body any way that they could, and since the digestive system was blocked, the skin was an avenue to get rid of some toxins. Acne was the result. Working to reduce toxins in your environment and in your food will help you to start the process of eliminating them from your body. The Optimal Mental Health Nutrition Plan helps you to eliminate toxins from your food. Begin now to reduce or eliminate the toxins in your everyday environment as much as possible. This includes the products you use on your body and hair as well as the products you clean with. There are many great products out there and many that you can easily make yourself. You will more specifically address toxicity in Phase Four of the program. It is important to have a healthy foundation before doing any kind of detoxification program.

Digestive Problems

While you sleep, the digestive system rests. If you eat a large meal before bed or have a lot of food in your system that is not properly digesting, it can impact your ability to sleep well. Working on healing the digestive tract can be very beneficial to improving sleep.

Food Sensitivities

If you have sensitivity to a food and you eat it during the day it can disrupt sleep. The most common food allergens are wheat, dairy, corn, nuts, and soy. These foods are removed in Phase One of the program. You may notice that your sleep has improved just by keeping these foods out of your diet. If you have other food sensitivities it will benefit you to keep these out of your diet as you work to heal the digestive tract. Take a look at your Food/Mood Log to help you determine if other foods may be problematic for you and eliminate them from your diet. This may be all you need to get a better nights rest. As you work on healing your digestive tract you may be able to add these foods back in at a later date.

Magnesium Deficiency

Magnesium is a mineral that helps to relax muscles. Magnesium deficiency can result in constipation, headaches, muscle tightness/spasms, and difficulty sleeping. If you have multiple symptoms of magnesium deficiency you may want to try taking 400 mg of magnesium before bed. This can be increased up to 1200 mg in a day. Increase slowly and pay attention to your stool. If you get too much magnesium you will have diarrhea. Increase until stool becomes loose then reduce your dosage. The product I have recommended the most for magnesium is Professional Complimentary Health Formulas Magnesium Complex. You will need to contact a qualified Nutritional Practitioner in order to purchase this product. Go to **www.GetAtTheRoots.com** to locate a Nutritional Practitioner near you.

Stress

Stress impacts the body and the brain. When the mind is unable to shut off it makes it difficult to fall asleep and stay asleep. There are multiple things you can do to help relieve stress, including the following:

1. Write down whatever is going through your mind to get it out of your mind and on paper.
2. Do not watch/read anything overly stimulating prior to bedtime.
3. Turn off the TV. Preferably do not have a TV in your bedroom.
4. Engage in activities that you enjoy daily.
5. Get outside help from a life coach or therapist.
6. Healthy relationships help to minimize stress. Surround yourself with positive people.

Phase Two Step Two: Healthy Sleep Review
✓ Keep blood sugar stable
✓ Reduce/eliminate toxins in your environment, health care products, cleaning products, etc.
✓ Continue to work on optimizing digestion and healing the digestive tract
✓ Determine and remove all food allergens/sensitivities
✓ Consider supplementing with Magnesium if you have symptoms of deficiency
✓ Work on things to reduce/eliminate stress

Chapter 12

Optimal Mental Health Nutrition Plan
Phase Three: Liver Health

"One of the basic tenets of naturopathic medicine is that many diseases can be treated by enhancing liver function." 7 Day Detox Miracle [1]

The liver is one of the largest organs in the body, and is responsible for over 500 functions within the body. It is absolutely vital that this organ is functioning well in order to obtain optimal mental and physical wellness. If your liver is in distress, you may feel tired, sluggish, could have headaches, dark circles under your eyes, and may suffer from depression, among other potential symptoms. In fact, liver disease is associated with both major depression and suicide attempts among adults.[2] This isn't to say you have to be diagnosed with liver disease to have a liver that is not functioning optimally. When the liver is not functioning optimally, there will be challenges to reaching optimal wellness. However, the liver has an amazing ability to regenerate itself and so, even if it is not functioning well, you can begin to nourish your liver and bring life and health back to it. Let's first talk about some of the roles of the liver that will impact your ability to obtain optimal mental wellness.

The Liver – the Body's Toxin Filter

One of the main roles of the liver is to filter toxins from the body. All blood is sent to the liver to be filtered to separate the beneficial components from the toxins such as bacteria, pesticides, medications, used hormones, etc. It is here that the liver then takes these substances through a two-step process of transforming the toxin into a form that can be removed from the body. These are known as Phase One and Phase Two detoxification pathways. It is quite a bit more complex than I will explain here, as I will attempt to keep things simple. In Phase One detoxification, the body uses enzymes to break down the toxin. This process results in the production of free radicals, and so antioxidants are needed in this phase to prevent damage. Chemical reactions occur to transform the toxin into a form that is then able to be removed once it is ready for Phase Two. This process of transforming the toxin in Phase One, however, leaves the substance in a more toxic form to the body and also potentially creates free radical damage if antioxidants are in short supply. Because of this, it is vitally important that both phases are supported with plenty of nutrition, so that the body does not become more toxic in the process. If the body is healthy and well-equipped nutritionally, to complete Phase One and Phase Two detoxification, then the toxins will successfully be removed from the body, as long as the digestive system is eliminating properly. Specific nutrients are needed for both phases of detoxification.

In order to support both Phase One and Phase Two detoxification pathways, you will want to be sure to supply the body with plenty of the foods rich in the nutrients needed to supply these pathways. It is also important that the digestive tract is properly eliminating so that, when the liver processes these toxins and dumps them into the colon, it is able to get them out of the body. If the body is not properly eliminating, you can cause a back-up of toxins in the body which may then be reabsorbed, making the body sicker. You have been preparing the body with the first eight weeks of the Optimal Mental Health Nutrition Plan to be able to now focus on maximizing the health of the liver. The digestive tract was addressed first, in order to set the stage for the liver to be able to remove these toxins from the body successfully, and optimize health in the body.

Phase One detoxification requires multiple B-vitamins, fat-soluble vitamins, essential fatty acids, antioxidants, and glutathione. The foods to help you to optimize these nutrients include fruits and root vegetables (beets and carrots are especially healthful to the liver), and healthy seafood. The body makes glutathione with the help from amino acids from protein foods and foods rich in sulfur. Exercise has been shown to increase glutathione, as well as improve liver health; however, over-exercising can have a detrimental effect on both. [1,3,4]

Phase Two detoxification requires multiple amino acids and sulfur. This is another reason why protein is vital to the body, as it is needed in the detoxification process. If amino acids are not properly supplied through protein in the diet, then Phase Two detoxification can be hindered resulting in a back-up of toxins in the body. Remember that Phase One left the toxin in a more toxic form, and so it is very important that the body is able to complete the process of detoxification with Phase Two, in order to be able to successfully remove the toxin. This is one reason I am not a fan of doing just juice fasts or water fasts in attempts to detox the body. Doing this does not supply the body with adequate nutrition to complete both phases of detoxification. Amino acids from protein foods are what are most needed for this. Be sure to eat plenty of healthy meats, fish, eggs, and broth in order to supply the body with what is needed to accomplish this. Sulfur rich foods are also needed for Phase Two detoxification. Foods rich in sulfur include the cruciferous vegetables (cabbage, broccoli, cauliflower), garlic, and onions. Drinking lemon water, particularly first thing in the morning, can also aid the liver in cleansing toxins.

It is also very important to support the health of the gallbladder. Let's review the role of the gallbladder. The gallbladder holds bile that was produced in the liver, and is released when needed to emulsify the fat in the diet. It also ushers toxins out of the body, via the digestive tract. Therefore, it is important that the gallbladder is functioning well. Foods to support a healthy gallbladder are raw beets, apples, and carrots. Turmeric and bitter vegetables such as dandelion greens, mustard greens, and chicory also help to stimulate bile.

The Liver's Stored Nutrients

The liver converts nutrients in our diet, and stores these nutrients to be released when needed by the body. The liver stores fat-soluble vitamins A, D, E, K, vitamin B12, iron, and copper, to be used by the body when needed as well as glycogen (from carbohydrates) for energy. Multiple nutrients are needed in the detoxification process and are also needed to supply the organs and tissues of the body. If the liver is overworked due to a high toxin load, it will not be able to adequately store and supply the body with the nutrients it needs to function optimally.

The Liver Produces Cholesterol & Bile

The liver is also responsible for producing both cholesterol and bile. Cholesterol makes up 50% of every cell membrane and, therefore, is essential for the health of the cells. We are made up of trillions of cells which comprise our organs and tissues and every part of our body. The health of the cells, therefore, dictates the health of our body. It is important that the cell membrane is healthy in order to function optimally. Cholesterol is needed to provide that healthy cell wall. Cholesterol is also needed to manufacture hormones. Without adequate cholesterol hormones will be in short supply. The liver not only removes the used hormones, but is also responsible for helping to make new hormones to be used by the body. If it is unable to properly get rid of the used hormones, as well as create the building blocks for the production of new hormones, then hormonal balance will be compromised. The next phase of the Optimal Mental Health Nutrition Plan will address hormone health. A healthy liver sets the stage for hormone balance.

The liver produces bile from cholesterol, bilirubin, and lecithin. It then stores it in the gallbladder to be released when there is fat in the meal, in order to break down the fat into components that can be used by the body. Bile also ushers toxins out of the body once the liver has broken them down. We've already learned how healthy fats are vital to optimal mental health, and bile is needed to obtain those benefits.

Nutrition and the Liver

The Optimal Mental Health Nutrition Plan sets the stage to begin assisting the liver in being able to detox successfully, by providing nourishing foods, helping to balance blood sugar through the foods eaten, hydrating the body to assist detoxification, and optimizing digestive health. Foods that are detrimental to the liver have been removed, such as sugar, alcohol, and bad fats. Although you will likely have these in your diet on occasion, it will be the exception instead of the rule. Eating a diet that helps to provide the nutrients needed for both Phase One and Phase Two detoxification, will prepare the body to successfully get rid of toxins, and thus promote a healthy body and mind.

Eating liver for the health of your liver

One of the best ways to nourish your liver is by eating a healthy liver organ from a healthy animal. You will want to choose liver from an animal that has been treated well, gets sufficient exercise, and has a healthy diet free of toxins. You will want liver from an animal that has not been given hormones or antibiotics. This is important, as we know that the liver filters toxins from the body. For that reason, you will want to choose a liver from an animal that has not had to filter hormones or antibiotics given to them. You can choose to eat liver from different animals such as a cow, chicken, turkey, deer, lamb, or any other animal that is healthy. Eating liver from an animal that is properly fed and raised will benefit your liver. If you do not like the taste of liver, there are recipes out there that can mask the taste. Chicken liver has a milder taste than beef liver. You can also opt to take a glandular supplement made from a healthy animal's liver. Eating liver two to four times per month is a great goal to have in keeping your liver healthy.

Not Feeling Well with Liver-Loving Foods?

If you don't feel well when you eat garlic and onions, it is potentially a sign that you are toxic, have a bacterial imbalance in the body, or a sluggish bowel. These foods are highly anti-bacterial, and help to kill off bad bacteria within the body. If there is an imbalance in the body, it can cause a detox response as the bad bacteria are eliminated. If the bowels are not functioning regularly to eliminate these toxins from the body, you can become more toxic and not feel well. These foods are helpful with detoxification and maintaining a healthy microbiome, but need to be introduced at the proper time and amounts, to ease the process and maximize success in obtaining health in the colon, liver, and body in general. This is also very important for optimal mental wellness, as detox reactions can have a negative impact mentally. Detoxification has to happen in the proper timing, and needs to be done gradually in order to maintain mental wellness in the process.

MY STORY: *I did not feel well when I ate garlic and onions and, in fact, I thought that I hated those foods. I also did not fare well with fermented foods either. I just didn't feel good after I ate them. I didn't understand at the time why that was; I just thought they were not good for me. That was the furthest thing from the truth. I desperately needed these foods in my body; however, I needed my body to be functioning well to handle the powerful benefits of those foods. Garlic, onions, and fermented foods all have a common benefit, and that is to destroy bad bacteria and provide an environment for the flourishing of good bacteria within the digestive tract. If there is an overgrowth of bad bacteria in the digestive tract, when you eat these foods, you create an environment for war within the gut. The die-off reaction creates toxins in the digestive tract that need to then be eliminated from the body. This is something that my body needed; however, my digestion was so sluggish that I became more toxic, as I was unable to eliminate frequently enough. When I was able to restore digestion and get my bowels moving regularly, I was able to eat and enjoy these foods without any negative effects. This required slowly introducing them at first, while I worked to create a healthy intestinal microbiome.*

It's also important to consider if you have supplied the body with the nutrients needed for Phase One detoxification, but it is lacking the nutrients needed for Phase Two, you will make yourself more toxic. Be sure that the bowels are moving regularly, and include foods to support both Phase One and Phase Two detoxification for optimal results.

Review – Liver Health

Nutrients to support liver & detoxification	
Antioxidants	Fruit, dark leafy greens, beets, carrots, milk thistle, lemon, turmeric
Glutathione	Sulfur-rich foods, amino acids, organ meats, healthy exercise all increase glutathione production by the body
Sulfur	Broccoli, cabbage, cauliflower, kale, Brussels sprouts, garlic, onion, radishes
Amino Acids	Healthy animal meats, liver, fish, eggs, and broth
Nutrients to support a healthy gallbladder	
Bitter vegetables	Dandelion greens, mustard greens, and chicory
Stimulate bile	Beets, artichoke, sauerkraut, ginger, apples, celery, lemon, radishes [5]
Healthy Fats	Avocados, olive oil

Chapter 13

Optimal Mental Health Nutrition Plan
Phase Four:
Step 1 – Hormone Health

When hormones are properly balanced, there is harmony within the body and we feel good. This has a direct effect on our mental well-being. In order to obtain optimal mental health, it is important to address hormone health. Now that you have built a solid nutritional foundation, you are ready to work on your hormones. The dietary plan is designed to support hormones naturally; however, if additional support is needed, then you will want to follow the guidelines in this chapter. An important component to helping recover hormonal balance is to identify the weak link.

Most women would probably agree to the fact that they know when their hormones are off balance, since they have learned the fluctuations that occur throughout their cycle each month. When their hormones are off, so is their mood. They may feel irritable, anxious, and/or depressed. Ask any of their significant others, and they will likely agree to this. So, with regards to female hormone fluctuations, it is easy for us to see the correlation between imbalanced hormones and imbalanced brain chemistry. So what about men? Men also need their hormones to be properly balanced in order to feel optimally well. For example, low testosterone can cause depression, and low progesterone can cause anxiety in men. So it is important to both men and women that hormones are in the proper balance. We often think of the sex hormones when we talk about hormone balance, but we need to consider that it is the balancing of all of our hormones that really creates harmony in the body. This chapter will cover the sex, adrenal, and thyroid hormones, as they are all important for optimal mental wellness.

The Optimal Mental Health Nutrition Plan encourages the foods needed for hormonal balance, such as healthy fats, cholesterol, and protein. If, after following the Nutrition Plan to Optimize Mental Health for a minimum of eight weeks, you are still having difficulty with imbalanced hormones, you will want to identify your weak link. Unbalanced hormones can be identified by a Naturopathic Physician through testing, and can be helpful in pinpointing your weak link.

WEAK LINK #1: Overburdened Liver

We are fighting a war of toxins in our world that is messing with our hormones: endocrine disruptors from food, pesticides, hormones and antibiotics in our meat, and BPA in our plastics and canned food liners. This is all wreaking havoc on our hormones and on our health in general. Let's address soy in our food first. Soy is an estrogen mimicker, and can disrupt our hormone balance. If you want to learn more about the dangers of soy, research the Weston A. Price Foundation and soy (**www.westonaprice.org**). You will find multitudes of studies listed, showing the dangerous effects of consuming soy on the health of the body. There has been a tremendous amount of research done to show soy's detrimental effect on health and, in particular, our hormones. Once touted as a health food, it is now being shown to be detrimental. The benefits of soy may come when that soy is fermented. However; the soy we are consuming is not often fermented, but is largely genetically modified. For this reason, the Optimal Mental Health Nutrition Plan eliminates soy altogether from your diet. Eating fermented soy on occasion is acceptable but, apart from that, you should endeavor to avoid it. Here is just some of what the research is showing us. Soy has been shown to cause enlargement of breasts in males,[1,2] decreased libido,[3] has been linked to breast cancer,[4] and may be a factor in infertility.[5] It's evident that soy has an effect on our hormones, and not in a good way.[6] Unfortunately, soy is used in many baby formulas, and research has shown that those who were given soy formulas as infants had more reproductive problems as adults.[7] Besides soy, other foods we are eating can impact our hormone balance within our body, such as foods that have been sprayed with pesticides, meats that are loaded with hormones and antibiotics, as well as food and drinks that have been contaminated with chemicals, such as BPA (Bis-phenol A), from the plastics that they are being stored in. These are all reasons to stick to nutritious organic foods, and avoid storing food or drinks in plastic. This is important if you want to obtain hormone balance and optimal mental wellness.

The health of the liver was addressed in the last phase, but will be discussed here, since it pertains to hormones in the body. The liver is responsible for detoxing those endocrine disruptors we just discussed, getting rid of hormones once they have accomplished their job, converting thyroid hormone T4 to T3 (more active form), assisting the body in maintaining blood sugar levels, and producing cholesterol (an essential component of hormone production). This can all impact the body's ability to maintain healthy hormones (sex hormones, thyroid, and adrenal hormones).

The liver breaks down hormones in the body once they have accomplished the job they were sent out to do. If, however, the liver is overburdened from toxins in the body, it is unable to properly metabolize these hormones, resulting in excess hormones in circulation. If the body is overburdened with toxins, it can hinder its ability to make cholesterol. Cholesterol is needed to make hormones; thus hormone production can be hindered. Therefore, it is important to address the health of your liver when hormonal imbalance is present.

Your liver has the ability to regenerate itself, and so you can improve the health of your liver by reducing burdens to the liver and then eating in a way as to bring nourishment and health to it, as was discussed in the previous chapter. Below is a quick review of ways to reduce the burden, as well as how to nourish your liver. It is important to follow these guidelines to optimize the health of your liver in order to assist the body in balancing hormones. Review Phase Three: Liver Health to optimize your success with hormones.

Reducing the burden to your liver
- ✓ Avoid sugar, alcohol, and bad fats (hydrogenated, partially hydrogenated oils, and trans-fats)
- ✓ Reduce/Eliminate toxins you are exposed to in your food, cleaning products, health care products, etc.

Nourishing your liver
- ✓ Eat dark leafy greens daily (including dandelion greens to optimize liver health)
- ✓ Include liver from a healthy animal in your diet, weekly. Take a liver glandular supplement if you have an aversion to organ meats. There are many healthy and tasty liver recipes you can try
- ✓ Eat foods daily to nourish the gallbladder such as raw beets, apples, and ginger.

WEAK LINK #2:
Hypothalamus Pituitary Communication

The hypothalamus communicates with the pituitary gland, which then sends messages to the gonads (HPG axis), as well as the adrenals (HPA axis), to increase or decrease hormones in order to maintain balance. The hormones work on a feedback loop, sending messages back to the pituitary gland, which then relays messages to the hypothalamus. Based on these signals, the hypothalamus instructs an increase or decrease in different hormones in order to maintain proper harmony in the body. If the communication between the hypothalamus and pituitary gland is disrupted, hormonal imbalance occurs.

Multiple things can cause interference in the communication between the hypothalamus and the pituitary gland. Here is a list of some things that can cause disruption in this very important communication system.

Causes of Disruption of HP (Hypothalamus-Pituitary) Communication:

- ✓ Medications – birth control, steroids, and others
- ✓ Stress
- ✓ Over-exercising
- ✓ Endocrine disruptors (pesticides, plastics, cleaners, etc.)
- ✓ Eating soy (an estrogen mimicker)

In order to restore the HPG (Hypothalamus-Pituitary-Gonad) & HPA (Hypothalamus-Pituitary-Adrenal) axis communication, it is important to reduce/eliminate the disrupters listed above. It can also be very effective in nourishing the hypothalamus and pituitary gland, by supporting them with a glandular supplement such as lamb pituitary and hypothalamus. Nourishing our organs by eating the organ of a healthy animal can be very helpful to restoring health to that organ. This can be done by taking glandular supplements when the actual organ is not available or not appealing to eat.

Restoring Hypothalamus Pituitary (HP) Communication:
- ✓ Reducing/eliminating disruptors listed above
- ✓ Taking a hypothalamus/pituitary gland supplement

MY STORY: *After moving into an older home, I quickly noticed I was not feeling myself. I had a really hard time concentrating, my energy was fading fast, and I started to break out in a rash. The rash eventually covered a good portion of my body, and itched terribly. I stayed in the home for one month before the symptoms became so bad that I was certain there was something in the house. I suspected mold. It was later discovered that the house was, in fact, infested with mold. After attempting to resolve my itchy rash and regain my energy through my diet, I was not getting far, even though I had removed myself from the environment. I eventually succumbed to prednisone and then a cortisone shot in order to finally take the edge off of the horrible itching. It still took six months before the itching completely went away, but it did wonders for the rash. As a result of taking the medication, my previously regular menstrual cycle went from a 28-day cycle to every other week. Recognizing that my HPG axis was not properly functioning, I began supplementing with a hypothalamus and pituitary glandular. After a month of supplementation, my cycle went back to its normal 28 days. I also had to restore bacterial balance in my body that was disrupted by the medication. These are things that need to be considered when you have taken or are taking medications of any kind. They can cause imbalances in the body that result in other problems arising.*

I have also had the opportunity to work with others to restore their hypothalamus pituitary communication, and thus restore health to the sex organs, as well as adrenals. One woman I worked with was not getting her period, and we discovered that it was due to stress and over-exercising that disrupted the HP axis. Supporting the hypothalamus and pituitary through glandular supplementation for a month, as well as reducing exercise, resulted in the restoration of her monthly cycle.

If the hypothalamus and pituitary gland are functioning properly, then you will want to look at what other links may be weak in order to resolve your hormone imbalance.

WEAK LINK #3: Overworked Adrenals

The adrenals are vital to the health of the body and are our "emergency" stress glands. Due to the overwhelming burden of stress in most people's lives these days, many people are experiencing a degree of adrenal fatigue. Your adrenal glands sit above your kidneys, and produce several adrenal hormones including Epinephrine (Adrenaline), Norepinephrine (Noradrenalin), Cortisol, DHEA, Pregnenolone, Progesterone, Estrogen, Testosterone, Androstenedione, and Aldosterone. Whenever your body is in a stressed state (emergency), the adrenals will secrete hormones (adrenalin and noradrenalin), slowing blood flow to organs of digestion and memory, and sending it to the working muscles. This is your fight or flight response. When your blood sugar drops too low, cortisol is released to tell the liver and muscles to release stored glycogen, and to break down protein if need be. Cortisol is also a powerful anti-inflammatory and central nervous system stimulator. Aldosterone is needed for the regulation of sodium and potassium. Whenever your body is in danger, your adrenal hormones will be secreted to allow your body to fight or run. However, because many of us live in a chronic state of stress, we are often signaling our adrenals, even though we are not in any real danger. Besides stress, some of the things that are causing our adrenals to be overworked are poor diet, blood sugar instability, over-exercising, and a lack of sleep. In order to obtain hormone balance in the body, you will need to identify whether your adrenals are a weak link for you. Here are some signs that your adrenals are struggling:

Eating fruit in the morning makes you shaky. Fruit is high in sugar and potassium. Potassium and sodium need to be properly balanced. When one is high, it depletes the other. So if potassium is high, it causes a reduction in sodium. The adrenals need sodium to function properly, and many people with suffering adrenals will crave salt as a result. Including sea vegetables and plenty of sea salt with your foods can help tremendously with this. Those whose adrenals are suffering a lot will do well to drink water with sea salt first thing in the morning, and should steer clear of fruit and high glycemic carbs at this time of the day. Choose a high protein, high fat, low-glycemic carb meal for breakfast.

Low Blood Sugar – Blood sugar levels greatly impact the adrenals. Just as it is a danger to your body for the blood sugar to stay elevated too long, it is also a danger if the blood sugar drops too low. If the blood sugar drops too low, it could lead to a coma and possibly death. However, before this happens, the adrenals (your emergency glands) will secrete cortisol. Cortisol tells your liver to release the stored sugar (glycogen) to elevate the blood sugar. Both high and low cortisol levels have been associated with major depression. [8,9] In order to prevent this stress on the body and subsequent release of adrenal hormones, you will want to eat a diet that will keep the blood sugar stable by following the base diet for the Optimal Mental Health Nutrition Plan, as well as exercising at a low to moderate intensity and properly fueling the body with healthy nutrients to keep blood sugar stable and nourish the adrenals.

Extreme fatigue - Everyday tasks have become more and more difficult. When your adrenals are fatigued, you will be, too.

Crave salt - Your adrenals need sodium to function properly, and are responsible for maintaining a balance between potassium and sodium. Individuals with adrenal fatigue often crave salt, as they tend be tipped towards higher potassium and lower sodium. Adding sea salt, which is rich in minerals, to your foods is a great way to keep proper balance in these minerals.

Dizzy when standing - Many people with low-functioning adrenals also have low blood pressure. This makes it difficult to get the blood pumping enough to get to the brain when going from a lying to a standing position. Therefore, you may feel dizzy when standing if your adrenals are overworked.

Memory problems - The adrenals are our stress glands, designed to come to our rescue in the event of an emergency. When the body's stress signals are triggered, they will hinder blood flow to digestion and to the parts of the brain responsible for memory, in order to send as much nutrients and sugar to the working muscles, so that you can fight the danger or run from the danger. This hinders digestion and also impacts memory. Therefore, stress impacts your ability to remember things. It is very important to focus on minimizing the stress response in your body, by keeping it well-nourished and taking time to rest and practice stress-relieving activities. This will do wonders for your adrenals.

Needing to wear sunglasses - When the adrenals are functioning properly, they are responsible for constricting your pupils when out in bright light. However, if the adrenals are overworked, they will have difficulty doing this. One of the tests for determining the level of adrenal fatigue in the body is the Paradoxical Pupillary Response Test. This test measures the response of the pupils (whether they constrict and stay constricted) with light. An individual who is suffering from adrenal fatigue will find it difficult to be outside in the sun without wearing shades.

MY STORY: *Through my journey of working to stabilize my blood sugar and identify the foods that were causing me trouble and get well, I experienced adrenal fatigue. It had become more and more difficult to do everyday tasks. Even blow-drying my hair had become a chore. I also would get dizzy upon standing. I can't count the number of times I stood up and my vision went black. It would typically not last long, and I would immediately sit down until my blood pressure was able to get blood to my brain, and my vision would quickly return. It was so bad at times that even squatting down to spot my clients when they were lifting weights and then standing back up caused me to get light headed and start to lose my vision. I never told my clients this was happening, but it was a real problem. Sometimes it would happen several times in one training session. On top of that, my memory was really bad. Growing up, I had an impeccable memory. I won several contests memorizing scripture. I did not like history in school, but I got mostly A's because, right before the test, I could memorize just about everything. My point is that I was young (early to mid-twenties) when this was happening. It shouldn't have been. Sometimes it was so bad when I was training clients that I would forget what exercises we had just done. It's a good thing I had an outline to remind myself what I had planned for the day with that particular client, even though I was known to create workouts on the spot and change things up constantly. So many times I would go to check out my client, when they had to sign off on their session, and I could not remember their name for the life of me. These were clients I had worked with for years. I never let on to them that this was happening. Again, it was good that I had their file handy and I could glance at it to remember their name. I also* *experienced coming out of a store and not remembering where I parked. I had to carry food with me in the event my blood sugar dropped. I would monitor my blood sugar occasionally to find it dropping sometimes within an hour of eating. This happened several times while I was out and I would find myself in stores unable to figure out what to do. I couldn't make a decision and had a hard time getting out of the store. I learned to know the signals and drop anything I was going to buy and get out of the store as soon as possible and get food in me. Keeping my blood sugar stable was essential, so I had food on me at all times. I had real trouble stabilizing my blood sugar. My sleep was also being affected. Many times my blood sugar would drop in the night; I would awaken and then cook myself a meal at 2 am. This was not a great way to live. It made it difficult to make plans and it left me totally exhausted. Restoring my adrenals was key to helping me get my blood sugar back in balance. Learning how to combine my foods was absolutely instrumental in helping me to stabilize my blood sugar. Getting my digestion, liver, and adrenals healthy was essential as well. This took time, as stress plays a major role in the health of the adrenals. I was certainly overstressed by all that was happening in my body and mind, but I was determined that I was going to get on the other side of this. It certainly took time, as I was figuring things out, but I am so grateful that I was able to restore my adrenals, as well as my mental health. Remember that stable blood sugar helps to keep energy and mood stable, which are both key to optimizing mental health. Keep on going; there is hope!*

The adrenal glands take time to recover, and you will need to nourish them and allow them to rest in order to accomplish this. Every time you tax the adrenal glands, according to James Wilson, author of *Adrenal Fatigue: The 21st Century Stress Syndrome*, it takes your body approximately 24-48 hours to recover.[10] How many people, after they tax their adrenals with a stressful moment at work, allow their bodies to rest for 24-48 hours? What happens is that we accumulate hours of time that our adrenals need to completely recover. If we do not give our body rest and allow the adrenals to restore, they get taxed further and further, leading to adrenal fatigue and eventual exhaustion. When the adrenals are functioning well, we feel on top of the world! We can do anything. We can stay up all night without effect. We are, however, taxing our adrenals while we do this and, over time, they will begin to fatigue. It is hard to tell someone at that moment that they need to slow down, because they feel great. Once their adrenals are stressed enough, they will begin to feel worse and worse, with less and less energy to do everyday tasks. I encourage you to find things you enjoy doing, and incorporate them into your life on at least a weekly basis – if not more. I encourage you to relax your body when you take a break at work, shut off your mind to the work at hand, and give your body and adrenals time to recover. It all adds up, and is absolutely essential to your recovery. If you do not allow your body to rest, eventually your body will force you to rest.

Guidelines to Restoring Adrenals
Healthy Living Guidelines

- ✓ Get plenty of rest – sleep is vital to the recovery of the adrenals
- ✓ Healthy exercise
- ✓ Sunshine
- ✓ Reduce/eliminate stress
- ✓ Healthy relationships
- ✓ Healthy environment

Dietary Recommendations to Restore Adrenals

- ✓ Nutrient-rich diet (Optimal Mental Health Nutrition Plan)
- ✓ Keep blood sugar stable to avoid taxing the adrenals
- ✓ Avoid fruit in the morning
- ✓ Sea salt to taste
- ✓ Reduce/eliminate caffeine
- ✓ Avoid sugar, alcohol, and processed foods
- ✓ Consider taking an adrenal glandular supplement to support the adrenals

WEAK LINK #4: Thyroid Dysfunction

The thyroid gland lies just below your Adam's apple in your neck. The thyroid gland produces three hormones; triiodothyronine (T3), thyroxine (T4), and calcitonin (which regulates blood calcium). The thyroid hormones control many body functions in the body, such as temperature regulation, growth and development, and metabolism.

Dysfunction of the thyroid impacts mental health. Some of the symptoms of thyroid dysfunction are also symptoms of mental illness, and sometimes hypothyroidism is wrongfully diagnosed as mental illness. Remember that mental illness is diagnosed based on a list of symptoms. There are root issues to those symptoms that are many times not discovered, but need to be adequately addressed and corrected. The thyroid is one of those areas that some physicians will look into when depression is present. Here is a list of some of the potential symptoms of hypo- and hyperthyroidism.

Symptoms of hypothyroidism: cold hands/feet, constipation, fatigue, difficulty concentrating, dry skin, low libido, slow heart rate, depression.

Symptoms of hyperthyroidism: Nervousness, irritability, fatigue, insomnia, racing heart, sweating, weight loss, hair loss, trembling.

Foods to Optimize Thyroid Health

Healthy cholesterol, fats, and protein are needed to manufacture all hormones, including your thyroid hormones. Thyroid hormones, T3 and T4, are composed of the amino acid tyrosine and iodine. As a result, it is important that the body is getting adequate nutrition in order to have the raw materials (tyrosine and iodine, along with other nutrients) needed to manufacture these hormones. Because of this, you will want to include foods that contain both iodine and tyrosine in your diet. Some examples of foods that are rich in iodine are sea vegetables, kelp, dulse, Himalayan sea salt, and cod. Some examples of foods that contain tyrosine are eggs, chicken, fish, shellfish, turkey, duck, pork, buffalo, ostrich, goat, veal, and spinach.

Foods that may hinder thyroid function

Goitrogenic foods suppress the thyroid and hinder its function. Soy is a goitrogen that has been shown to suppress the thyroid and slow metabolism.[11] We've already discussed how important staying away from soy is to hormone health, so this gives us even more reason. Other goitrogenic foods are not all bad, so you will want to look at the whole picture and limit these foods, but don't avoid them totally. Some examples of goitrogenic foods include: pine nuts, peanuts, millet, strawberries, pears, peaches, spinach, sweet potato, broccoli, cauliflower, radishes, cabbage, turnips, collard greens, and Brussels sprouts. Some of these foods are full of nutrients and helpful in supporting digestion and detoxification, so you will want to be sure to get a variety of vegetables in your diet and keep these foods in your diet, but limit their intake if your thyroid is not functioning optimally.

Consider the Health of the Adrenals

When looking at the health of the thyroid, one should always look at the health of the adrenals. They go hand in hand. In fact, treating hypothyroidism by treating adrenal insufficiency resulted in a reversal of hypothyroidism in three case studies.[12] It is important to minimize stress so that you do not overtax your adrenals, thus hindering thyroid function as well.

Toxins impact on the thyroid

The thyroid is impacted by toxins, particularly fluoride and chlorine. Both have been shown to suppress thyroid function.[13,14] For this reason, you will want to drink clean, filtered water free of these toxins, as well as filter your bathing water and choose a fluoride-free toothpaste.

Guidelines to Optimize Thyroid Function
Foods to Optimize Thyroid Function

- ✓ Tyrosine-rich foods: Sea vegetables, kelp, dulse, Himalayan sea salt, cod
- ✓ Iodine-rich foods: Eggs, chicken fish shellfish, turkey, duck, pork, buffalo, ostrich, goat, veal, spinach

Avoid/Limit these foods that hinder thyroid function

- ✓ Avoid soy
- ✓ Limit goitrogens: pine nuts, peanuts, millet, strawberries, pears, peaches, spinach, sweet potatoes, broccoli, cauliflower, radishes, cabbage, turnips, collard greens, Brussels sprouts

Other Considerations

- ✓ Filter water to avoid fluoride and chlorine
- ✓ Support the health of the adrenals to optimize thyroid function

✓ Consider taking a thyroid glandular supplement to support your thyroid

REVIEW: Hormone Balance

Nutritional Guidelines to Balance Hormones

1. Eat plenty of healthy protein, fats, and carbohydrates (this should already be established with the Base Dietary Plan and is essential to assisting your body in being able to properly balance hormones)

2. Eat healthy organ meats to assist the body in nourishing organs in the body. The liver is important, as it makes cholesterol which is needed to manufacture hormones. If the liver is overburdened, it will hinder its ability to create cholesterol and thus hinder hormone production.

3. Supplement with glandulars to support the hypothalamus, pituitary, sex glands, thyroid, and/or adrenals.

4. Supplement with fish oil to help assist the body in the production of hormones.

5. For those with adrenal fatigue, be sure to get adequate mineral-rich sea salt (limit this if you also have high blood pressure), avoid fruit in the morning, focus on keeping blood sugar stable, and get plenty of sunshine.

6. For those with thyroid dysfunction, minimize goitrogenic foods and eat foods rich in tyrosine and iodine to assist in thyroid hormone production.

Other Recommendations to Balance Hormones

1. Minimize stress. Stress impacts the adrenal glands and can wreak havoc on your hormones. Engaging in activities to bring joy into your life and minimize stress will benefit your hormones.
2. Sex within a healthy relationship helps to foster healthy hormones. However, this may be a cause of trauma for those who have experienced abuse, therefore having a detrimental impact. Getting help to heal from this is important to optimizing mental health.
3. Sleep is very important to the health of your hormones. Follow the guidelines from Phase Two to optimize sleep.

Chapter 14

Optimal Mental Health Nutrition Plan
Phase Four: Step 2 – Detoxification

MY STORY: *In my journey to find true freedom from mental illness, I was slowly uncovering, layer by layer, the root issues that were keeping me from being mentally well. It took me the longest to uncover one of my largest blocks to total freedom. That was heavy metal toxicity. This was revealed to me by multiple practitioners, but really didn't hit home until I met a Nutritional Therapy Practitioner who told me I was heavy metal toxic in arsenic, lead, and mercury, and that I wouldn't fully heal until I worked to remove these toxins from my body. I couldn't understand why I would be heavy metal toxic until I began to look into my upbringing. My mother was pregnant with me in 1976, and lived in Niagara Falls, NY not far from the Love Canal, which that year was discovered to be contaminated from a chemical spill. I also learned that the high school that I went to and played three sports a year at had a chemical waste dump directly behind it. Both of these were huge flags to why I was heavy metal toxic. That, coupled with the severe constipation for years, which did not allow my body to easily rid toxins, was a clear-cut reason why I could certainly be heavy metal toxic. This was the final key that I needed to help me truly obtain the health in my body and mind.*

Heavy Metal Toxicity

Heavy metals such as mercury, lead, arsenic, aluminum, and others can have a huge impact on mental wellness.[1-4] Heavy metals such as these have been shown to impact the nervous system, and multiple studies have been done to show the detrimental impact that these heavy metals have on the brain. Some of this research has shown that higher blood levels of lead are associated with an increased incidence of major depression and panic disorder.[5] A study was conducted on 526 men living in or near Boston, Massachusetts. These men had higher levels of lead in their blood and bone. The results showed a higher degree of anxiety, phobic anxiety, and depression among those with high lead levels.[6] Mercury damages the brain, kidneys, and lungs,[7] and exposure to arsenic is associated with neurologic problems.[8] As a result, each person should consider the possibility of heavy metal toxicity in your body contributing to mental health problems.

We are exposed to multiple toxins in our environment every day. Some people are exposed to more than others, based on where they live and work. We encounter toxins in the air we breathe, the water we drink and bathe in, the foods we eat (pesticides, hormones, antibiotics), our cleaning products, furniture, paint, and our skin and hair care products, among other things. Toxins are everywhere around us. We cannot completely eliminate toxins from our environment, but we can minimize the amount of toxins we are exposed to.

In order to reach optimal mental health, it is very important to minimize the toxins in your environment and eliminate toxins from your body. The Optimal Mental Health Nutrition Plan is designed to assist the body in detoxing. Amino acids from protein-rich foods are needed in the detoxification process, fiber from healthy organic produce helps to cleanse the body of toxins and keep the colon healthy, and healthy fats help to provide healthy cell walls that help protect cells from toxins. This sets the stage for the body to naturally eliminate toxins on a consistent basis. However, some of you may have an overabundance of toxins in your system, and may need additional help to further detoxify your body.

Potential Causes of Toxicity: Poor diet, pesticides, air and water pollution, household cleaners, amalgam fillings, medications/antibiotics, heavy metal exposure, problems with digestion and elimination, liver dysfunction, stress, and toxins in plastics.

How to determine if you are overloaded with toxins

Most people who are toxic feel it. I certainly did. I knew that I was toxic, and I tried many detox programs with no success. In fact, I felt much worse when I tried to detox. This helped me to understand the importance of preparing the body before beginning any kind of detoxification program. You may need to get professional assistance from a Nutritional Therapy Practitioner or Naturopathic Physician who is experienced with detoxification to assist you along the way. We are all exposed to toxins; however, consider the list below to determine if your body is not adequately able to remove toxins.

Check all the potential symptoms of toxin overload that apply to you:

- ☐ Body odor
- ☐ Skin conditions
- ☐ Edema
- ☐ Digestive problems
- ☐ Bad breath
- ☐ Cellulite
- ☐ Lymph node tenderness
- ☐ Headaches
- ☐ Pain
- ☐ Hormonal Imbalances
- ☐ Motion sickness
- ☐ Varicose veins
- ☐ Fatigue
- ☐ Puffy eyes or dark circles
- ☐ Difficulty concentrating
- ☐ Inflammation
- ☐ Chemical sensitivities
- ☐ Hemorrhoids
- ☐ Sleep problems
- ☐ Excess weight
- ☐ Sinus congestion
- ☐ Canker sore

Determining if you are overloaded with toxins

1. Are you experiencing symptoms of toxin overload?
   YES   NO

2. Have you been exposed to chemicals, heavy metals, air pollutants, etc. in your home, work, childhood, etc.?
   YES   NO

3. **Heavy Metal Urine Test** – You can opt to have a laboratory test your urine for the presence of heavy metals. However, these tests are not always accurate, depending on the amount of heavy metals circulating. If they are stored in the tissues, this test may not show them in the urine. I believe that this test is most accurate when a chelating agent is used prior to the collection of the urine, in order to draw the heavy metals out of the tissues. However, this can be dangerous as chelating agents can have side effects. If you are interested in getting a heavy metal urine test done, you will need to contact a Nutritional or Naturopathic Professional who has access to this testing and trained to assist in detoxification.

4. **Heavy Metal & Mineral Hair Analysis** – This can be an easy way to determine the level of minerals and toxicity in the body. This should also be done with the guidance of a Naturopathic Physician or Nutritional Therapy Practitioner trained in assessing mineral hair analysis tests.

STEPS TO DETOXING

Following these steps to detoxification will help you to optimize health and wellness when done at the appropriate times, when the body is ready. You know you are ready for further detoxification when your digestive system is eliminating regularly (1-3 normal bowel movements per day) and the kidneys and liver are healthy. Even while you are working to optimize the health of the digestive tract, kidneys, and liver you can begin to reduce/eliminate toxins in your environment as well as detox through the skin (steps 1 & 2 in the following section).

Our bodies eliminate toxins in many different ways through our body systems (cardiovascular system, digestive system, respiratory system, lymphatic system, urinary system, and the skin). Because the body eliminates toxins through various pathways, you will want to detoxify the body both externally and internally to optimize success.

It's important to prepare the body prior to doing a specific detox program. Just like it was important to gradually introduce bone broth and fermented foods, as well as to gradually reduce gluten, casein, and sugar, you want to minimize a detox reaction by properly preparing the body in advance. The dietary program has already laid the ground work to begin the process of both external and internal detoxification. If your foundations for mental health are still not properly functioning then you will need to go back and work further on them from chapters 6-12, prior to beginning a more intense detoxification program.

Step 1: Reduce/Eliminate Toxins

This step includes taking an inventory of the toxins that you are exposed to on a regular basis. You should at this point be consuming mostly organic foods free of pesticides, hormones, and antibiotics. You should also be drinking clean, filtered water from glass instead of plastic. It's important to store your food in glass and not plastic, in order to prevent the leaching of chemicals into your food. Next, take an inventory of what you are putting on your skin from shampoos, soaps, lotion, and make-up, and then transition to non-toxic products. Anything you put on your skin gets absorbed into your body so, if you can't eat it, it should not be put on your skin. I often use a combination of coconut oil, olive oil, hemp oil, and/or lavender oil on my skin. Next, consider what you are using to clean your home with. There are many things you can make at home. I mostly clean my home with baking soda and vinegar, which kills bacteria very effectively without causing any harm. A sick home will lead to sick people living in the home. Mold is very toxic to the body, and can be detrimental to your health. If you suspect that you have mold in your home you need to fully correct the problem or move. You will not be successful in reaching optimal mental wellness if you are living in a mold-infested home. Creating a home environment that is healthy is very important to your overall mental and physical health.

Step 2: External Detox

The skin is a major eliminating organ, and can assist the body in detoxifying while you work to prepare the body for internal detoxification. Exercising to the point of perspiration and sweating in a dry or far-infrared sauna are great ways to help eliminate toxins. Baths using Epsom salts, sea salt, or baking soda are great ways to assist the body in detoxifying as well. Other methods include ionic foot baths and clay baths. These methods help to draw toxins to the surface of your skin and pull them out of the body. While toxins are being eliminated through the skin, you may also lose minerals and so it is important to replenish those minerals. Green drinks that include things like spirulina, chlorella, and other green and sea vegetables are packed with minerals, nutrients, and amino acids to restore these to the body. Coconut water is another great way to replenish electrolytes.

Step 3: Internal Detox

It's important to talk about the lymphatic system when understanding detoxification. Our lymphatic system runs alongside our circulatory system in a similar fashion. The difference is that the circulatory system works as the heart continuously pumps blood throughout the body. The lymphatic system does not automatically pump but requires outside action to push the lymphatic fluids along. The lymphatic system is responsible for pulling the fluids including toxins and bacteria from tissues and collecting them in the lymph nodes where bacteria and viruses are attacked and then the fluids are returned to the circulatory system via vessels in the upper body. However, this requires action on our part. We need to move our lymphatic system in order to push the toxins through to then be eliminated. We do this through things such as exercise, massage, rebounding, and dry skin brushing. Although these actions are taking place externally, they are impacting what is happening internally with the lymphatic system as it pushes toxins out of the body.

It's important to continuously support the organs of detoxification in order to assist the body to optimize the success of eliminating toxins from the body. The lymphatic system pulls toxins from tissues and then returns that fluid to the circulatory system. The circulatory system takes all blood to the liver to filter toxins from the body, as we learned earlier. In review, both the liver and gallbladder help to assist the body in ridding toxins. Toxins are ushered to the liver to then be filtered, and then the toxins are removed from and ushered out of the body via bile that is released from the gallbladder. Although the Optimal Mental Health Nutrition Plan helps to improve the health of these digestion organs, some may need some additional support. Providing nutrition to these organs in the form of either herbal support or glandular support via supplementation or with the consumption of healthy liver from a healthy animal can be a great way to do this. Consuming healthy liver from a healthy animal on a regular basis can be a great way to ensure a healthy liver. Following a nutritional program to feed the organs of detoxification is important to do for a minimum of four weeks and up to several months before you would consider doing any specific detox program designed to draw more toxins that may be stored in the tissues.

Certain things can assist the body in removing heavy metals from the body. Magnesium binds to mercury, to then pull it out of the body. I believe this is one reason magnesium can be depleted easily in some individuals who have multiple amalgam fillings in their mouths as mercury vapors are constantly being released. Magnesium helps to bind them and pull them out, leaving less magnesium for the rest of the body. Magnesium is needed for optimal mental health and you will learn about the importance of magnesium in the next phase to determine if supplementation may be beneficial for you. Charcoal also helps to bind toxins to pull them out of the body. The key with charcoal is that the bowels need to be moving regularly so that, when the charcoal attracts the heavy metals, you are able to get them out of the body and they do not end up getting reabsorbed. Food-grade diatomaceous earth can absorb heavy metals, bacteria, viruses, and parasites in the body.[9] It's important to start very slowly (1/4 tsp.) then gradually increase to a heaping tbsp. Some individuals experience a detox response, and so you will want to test it out with a very small amount first. Other herbal remedies also assist the body in drawing more toxins from the tissues. Always keep in mind that if you are not moving your bowels regularly you are becoming more toxic. If bowels are not moving, you want to assist your body to get them moving through herbal or magnesium supplementation, while you work to get at the root of why the bowels are not eliminating regularly. However, it's important to assist the bowels in the process in order to avoid becoming more toxic.

Step 4: Seek Additional Help

If you have done all these things and you are still struggling with toxicity in your body, I would highly recommend getting professional help through a qualified Nutritional or Naturopathic Practitioner, who understands the importance of building healthy foundations and healthy digestion prior to completing any specific detox program.

Review: Detoxification	
Step 1: Reduce/Eliminate toxins in your everyday environment	Personal care products, cleaning products, water, eating clean
Step 2: External Detox	Sweating, Dry Far-Infrared Sauna, Baths (Epsom salt, sea salt, baking soda, or clay baths)
Step 3: Internal Detox	Exercise, massage, rebounding, dry skin brushing, nutrients to support liver, gallbladder, & kidneys. Pulling toxins out of the body.
Step 4: Professional Help	Seek Help from a Qualified Nutritional Practitioner to assist detox with an understanding of properly preparing the body prior to detox.

Chapter 15

Optimal Mental Health Nutrition Plan
Phase Five: Specific Nutrients

"The control of mental disease by varying the concentrations in the brain of nontoxic substances that are normally present, such as nicotinic acid and ascorbic acid, is preferred to the use of phenothiazenes and other means of therapy that involve a greater insult to the body and mind." Linus Pauling, 1967 Orthomolecular Psychiatry [23]

Bank of Nutrients

The Bank of Nutrients is a way of explaining how we are all different, based on the health of our bodies. Each person is born with a certain level of nutrients, so to speak, that we will call the bank of nutrients, based on the health of your parents, particularly your mother, when she carried you. The health of your mother and whether she was stressed, exposed to toxins, or had any other health issues or compromised systems of the body, impacted your health when you were born. Some are born with a healthy bank of nutrients, and others have a low bank of nutrients. This can be compared to a financial bank. Some have plenty of wealth and are able to cover all their expenses, whereas others are not making enough to cover expenses, and are feeling the pain of it. Just like more money in the bank helps to cover the expenses of living, and puts you in a place of security, financially-speaking, building health in a similar manner will result in a healthier, happier, more energetic future. You can do this by making more deposits into your bank of nutrients instead of withdrawals. So, what things result in a growing bank of nutrients versus a shrinking bank of nutrients? The table below lists some things that result in bank withdrawals and bank deposits.

Bank of Nutrients Chart

Bank Deposits	Bank Withdrawals
Nutrient-Dense Diet	Poor Diet
Healthy Digestion	Digestive Problems
Healthy Environment	Toxic Environment
Meditation/Prayer	Alcohol, Drugs
Healthy Relationships	Unhealthy Relationships
Healthy Nervous System	Vertebral Subluxations
Healthy Exercise	Over-Exercising
Laughter/Fun	Stress

As was already stated, each person starts with a certain level of nutrients in their bank, based largely on the health of their mother when she carried them. If an individual starts life out with a strong, high level of nutrition, they are less likely to see problems in their health initially. Over time, if they make too many withdrawals, they will begin to see deterioration in their health. The point where an individual begins to notice a negative change in health, in our example will be called the SYMPTOM LINE. I have often encountered clients who say that their symptoms cannot be due to a poor diet, because they have eaten that way for a long time, or even their whole lives, and they did not have symptoms until now. I explain the bank of nutrients, and that their poor diet, along with other things over time, have resulted in enough withdrawals that have pushed them beyond the symptom line, so that they are now experiencing symptoms. The table on the following page is an example of an individual who had a strong bank of nutrients with a nutrient-dense diet, lived and worked in a healthy environment, and exercised regularly, but began to show symptoms as a result of stress, poor digestion, and an unhealthy relationship. To help an individual in this instance, one would want to work on resolving the areas that are leading to withdrawals, and have them work on depositing more nutrients into their banks in order to build it up to a healthy level. An individual who is starting out with a low bank of nutrients will begin to show symptoms much sooner. That individual will require more building, or deposits, of nutrition in order to build a strong bank. This explains why some individuals will be able to obtain optimal mental health more quickly than others, based on their starting bank of nutrients, and some will require more super nutrition than others in order to reach optimal mental wellness.

An Example:

Bank of Nutrients
Unhealthy Relationship
Poor Digestion
Stress
Symptom Line
Exercise
Healthy Environment
Nutrient-Dense Diet

The term 'orthomolecular' was first coined by Nobel Prize-winner Linus Pauling, in which he defines it as "the provision of the optimum molecular environment for the mind." [24] Orthomolecular psychiatry identifies deficiencies and supplies the brain with the nutrition necessary to bring about optimal function. It is sometimes referred to as megavitamin therapy, as it works to provide super-nutrition (above the standard doses of nutrients) bringing health to the body and mind. There are many Orthomolecular Practitioners who focus their practices on providing therapeutic nutrition based on biochemical individuality (**www.orthomolecular.org**). Nutritional Therapy Practitioners, trained through the Nutritional Therapy Association, also work on creating plans based on biochemical individuality (**www.nutritionaltherapy.com**). Both are great resources if you are looking for additional support in identifying nutrient deficiencies and personally tailoring a supplement/nutrition program to correct for any imbalances. You can also go to **www.GetAtTheRoots.com** to find a qualified Nutritional Practitioner trained in the Get At The Roots Nutrition Program, designed to identify root issues hindering your ability to obtain optimal health and wellness.

In this phase, you will want to identify areas from which your nutrient bank is being depleted and work to build up your bank of nutrients. You may choose to have testing done to determine nutrient deficiencies and work from there, or you can identify potential deficiencies based on symptoms. Identifying your nutrient deficiencies will help to more quickly fine tune your program and optimize your nutrient bank.

Potential Tests to Determine Nutrient Deficiencies

Micronutrient Test for amino acids, multiple vitamins and minerals: (options: blood test; hair mineral analysis)

Essential Fatty Acid Profile: blood test for ratios of omega-3, 6, and 9 fats in the body.

Specific Nutrients to help boost brain chemistry

Research has shown the relationship between nutrient deficiencies and psychiatric illnesses.[1] Deficiencies can exacerbate symptoms of mental health, and so you will want to work to identify and correct any deficiencies when working to obtain optimal mental wellness. The following nutrients can influence mental health when deficiencies are present. While you can take supplements to support your diet, it is important to get as much nutrition as possible from the foods you eat. Listed here are potential deficiency symptoms and food sources of vitamins, minerals, and nutrients that are needed for optimal brain function.

- ✓ **B-vitamins** – Needed for energy and to manufacture your mood-enhancing neurotransmitters.
    - o **B1 (Thiamine)** helps with blood sugar control and can impact anxiety.
        - Deficiency Symptoms: Loss of appetite, depression, irritability, confusion, loss of memory, inability to concentrate, fear of impending doom, and sensitivity to noise.[2]
        - Food Sources: Fish, pork, nuts, seeds, lentils, beans, green peas, rice, acorn squash, asparagus[1,3]
    - o **B3 (Niacin)** is involved in many enzyme reactions and helps with the synthesis of serotonin.[1] Niacin has been shown to be helpful in the treatment of schizophrenia.[4] Deficiencies of niacin and vitamin C can lead to higher copper levels. Some individuals with schizophrenia and bipolar disorder have elevated copper levels.[5]

- Deficiency Symptoms: Anxiety, depression, fatigue [2]
- Food Sources: Fish, chicken, turkey, pork, lamb liver, beef, mushrooms, green peas, sunflower seeds, avocados [1]
- **B6 (Pyridoxine)** is important for protein metabolism, the nervous system, and immune system.
    - Deficiency Symptoms: Irritability, depression, confusion, abnormal EEG, seizures [7]
    - Food Sources: Sunflower seeds, pistachios, tuna, turkey, chicken, pork, beef, bananas, avocado, spinach [8]
- **B9 (Folate)** is needed for the synthesis of serotonin, dopamine, and epinephrine. [22]
    - Deficiency Symptoms: Diarrhea, depression, confusion, anemia [9]
    - Food Sources: Beans, lentils, spinach, asparagus, lettuce, avocado, broccoli, tropical fruits, oranges [10]
- **B12 (Cobalamin)** plays a key role in the nervous system and energy and can impact brain chemistry as a result.
    - Deficiency Symptoms: Poor concentration, anemia, fatigue, mania, depression, paranoia, agitation, delirium, confusion, long term can cause damage to nervous system and brain [2,11,12]
    - Food Sources: Clams, oysters, mussels, liver, fish, crab, beef, eggs [12]

✓ **Vitamin C** – Needed for the synthesis of serotonin and norepinephrine.[1] It is needed to create ATP, dopamine, peptide hormones, and tyrosine. [13] Vitamin C has been shown to be beneficial in high doses for those suffering from schizophrenia. [4]

- o Deficiency Symptoms: Mental weariness, lack of energy, weakness, irritability, weight loss [14]
- o Food Sources: Peppers, guavas, dark green leafy vegetables, kiwi, broccoli, berries, citrus fruits, tomatoes, peas, papaya [13]

✓ **Magnesium** – Magnesium is a natural relaxer. It helps with stress and is needed to manufacture brain chemistry. It's needed for healthy nerve and muscle function, and for many enzyme reactions in the body. [15] Magnesium supplementation is best taken at night as it helps to relax the body and enhance sleep.

- o Deficiency Symptoms: Muscle cramps, headaches, constipation, anxiety disorders, irregular heartbeat, insomnia
- o Food Sources: Dark leafy greens, nuts, seeds, fish, beans, lentils, avocados, bananas, dark chocolate. [15]

✓ **Vitamin D3** – Vitamin D is a hormone that impacts the release of neurotransmitters dopamine and serotonin.[16] Seasonal Affective Disorder impacts individuals during the winter seasons when there is less light and, hence, less natural vitamin D. Several studies have linked low vitamin D levels to depression.[16] Vitamin D is a fat soluble vitamin. When supplementing it needs to be taken with healthy fats in order to be absorbed in the body. Sunlight is a great source of vitamin D so get out into the sunshine to get your daily dose if possible.

- o Deficiency Symptoms: Muscle aches, muscle weakness, bone pain [17]
- o Food Sources: Cod liver oil, oily fish, mushrooms, caviar, pork, eggs [18]

- ✓ **Omega-3 Fats** – These can have a tremendous impact on mental health. Studies have shown great benefits to mood and brain function. [19] Some individuals will need more than others while working to build optimal mental health. The Harvard study that showed tremendous benefit to those suffering from bipolar disorder by supplementing with fish oil used nine grams of fish oil per day.[20] Keep this in mind, as some of you will require a higher dose than others while working to obtain mental wellness. As a reminder, fish oil is a natural blood thinner and so you will want to be careful when taking high doses. Contact your physician if you are currently taking any blood thinning medication or if you are undergoing surgery.
    - Deficiency Symptoms: Dry skin, fatigue, depression, achy joints, difficulty losing weight, memory problems, muscles easily fatigued, cravings for fatty foods, moodiness, irritability, tension headaches at the base of the skull
    - Food Sources: Fish oil, flaxseed oil, chia seeds, walnuts
- ✓ **Multiple Amino Acids** can have a positive impact on brain chemistry, but you will want to go to a Nutritional Practitioner to customize a program for you. Amino Acid supplementation may be contraindicated for certain mental illnesses, and so it is advised to seek professional help with someone trained in the field of amino acid therapy. [21] I personally did not fare well years ago when I attempted to use single amino acids to restore my brain chemistry. This is one reason I urge caution, even though there are some of you who may benefit tremendously.

It's important to note that certain medications can cause a deficiency in nutrients. As a result, if you are on medication, you may need additional nutrient support to compensate in order to reach optimal health and wellness.

Chapter 16
Building A Healthy Mind Through Fitness

Exercise is good for the body and brain. However, over-exercising is damaging to both the body and brain. Therefore, you need to find a happy medium and learn to listen to your body. God has created us so wonderfully, and equipped us with signals and indicators as to the health of our body. If we simply can get in tune with those signals we will be much better off physically and mentally. Pain is our body's way of telling us that something is wrong. We need to listen to those signals. If you are not currently exercising, begin slowly and listen to your body. Do not overdo it, and do not start doing higher intensity exercise if you are not currently. You may even need to reduce the intensity of your exercise if you are currently engaging in prolonged high-intensity exercise on a regular basis. When we over-exercise it sets out a host of stress signals in our body that cause the release of stress hormones. This cascade of hormones ultimately impacts our brain chemistry. Also, excessive exercise has been shown to cause an increase in the permeability of the digestive tract, which ultimately can have a negative impact via the gut-brain connection.[1]

Exercising at the appropriate intensity is good for the body and brain, and causes the release of your feel good hormones, your endorphins. A review of over 26 years of research on exercise and depression has shown its profound impact on not just treating depression, but also on the prevention of further relapses into depression. This occurred with moderate intensity and even low-intensity activities, such as gardening and walking for 20-30 minutes.[2,3] Other studies showed a mental health benefit from either 35 minutes of brisk walking, five times per week, or 60 minutes of brisk walking, three times per week. [4] These effects should be a motivating factor to include exercise in your schedule in order to optimize mental health.

Exercise is also beneficial, as it helps to assist the body in the detoxification process by moving the lymph. Exercise has positive benefits both physically and mentally, and should be incorporated into everyone's plan to reach optimal mental wellness. I recommend beginning very slowly and seeking professional help from a personal trainer (particularly if you are incorporating weight training) to be sure that you are properly exercising and using good form to avoid injury.

If you are currently not active, I would recommend beginning a low intensity exercise program, such as walking or biking, to get the body moving. Choose activities that you enjoy and gradually increase the time.

Beginner Exercise Program

Here is a sample beginner program that you may want to implement to optimize mental health:

Month One: Choose a low-intensity exercise such as walking, biking, or dancing. Activity should be done most days of the week, with a day of rest each week. I want to emphasize again the importance of listening to your body. If you feel you need to take more rest between exercise sessions or reduce the time you exercise that day, then it is best to listen to your body. However, if you simply do not feel like exercising, I would encourage finding a friend to be active with to keep you moving forward with your exercise. Choosing an activity that you enjoy will make it easier to continue on a regular basis.

Begin by walking/biking for 10 minutes, increase by two minutes every third day until you are active for a minimum of 30 minutes most days of the week. Listen to your body and increase more slowly if needed.

Day 1:	Walk/Bike	10 minutes
Day 2:	Walk/Bike	10 minutes
Day 3:	Walk/Bike	12 minutes
Day 4:	Walk/Bike	12 minutes
Day 5:	Walk/Bike	14 minutes
Day 6:	Walk/Bike	14 minutes
Day 7:	Rest	
Day 8:	Walk/Bike	16 minutes
Day 9:	Walk/Bike	16 minutes
Day 10:	Walk/Bike	18 minutes
Day 11:	Walk/Bike	18 minutes
Day 12:	Walk/Bike	20 minutes
Day 13:	Walk/Bike	20 minutes
Day 14:	Rest	
Day 15:	Walk/Bike	22 minutes
Day 16:	Walk/Bike	22 minutes
Day 17:	Walk/Bike	24 minutes
Day 18:	Walk/Bike	24 minutes
Day 19:	Walk/Bike	26 minutes
Day 20:	Walk/Bike	26 minutes
Day 21:	Rest	
Day 22:	Walk/Bike	28 minutes
Day 23:	Walk/Bike	28 minutes
Day 24:	Walk/Bike	30 minutes
Day 25:	Walk/Bike	30 minutes

It takes 21 days to form a habit. It's important to continue to exercise in order to create a habit, but always listen to your body and adjust the exercise in order to optimize your success in obtaining mental health.

Be sure to stretch all muscles at the end of your exercise session. This will help to prevent injury and reduce soreness and pain.

Month Two: Once you have established a fitness base with low-intensity exercise, then you may want to incorporate other forms of exercise to optimize success and your enjoyment with activity. It is recommended to find activities that you enjoy. Some options are as follows:

- Group Fitness Classes
- Weight Training
- Circuit Training
- Dance
- Biking
- Walking/jogging
- Hiking

Intermediate Exercise Program

For those who are currently active, continue to be active. However; you will want to consider the possibility that you may be over-exercising, which can hinder your ability to obtain optimal mental wellness. If you are exercising daily more than 1-1.5 hours, and you are not an athlete, you will want to consider decreasing your exercise and see how you feel. This will vary from person to person, but should be addressed. The goal is to be active three to six days of the week, at a low to moderate intensity for 20-60 minutes. This will vary per person and depend on your current level of fitness.

For those looking for a more personalized program, I highly recommend having a program designed for you by a qualified personal trainer. When choosing a trainer you will want to consider a few things. You will want to find out if the individual has a degree in the field such as exercise science, physiology, or athletic training. You will also want to find out if they have a certification and have maintained it. Some great certifications come from the National Strength and Conditioning Association (NSCA), American College of Sports Medicine (ACSM), Aerobics and Fitness Association of America (AFAA), and American Council on Exercise (ACE). There are several certifications out there that can be achieved with a few hours of training or by taking a test online. I don't encourage hiring someone with this little experience, but instead someone who has been certified by a reputable association and also one with experience.

Unfortunately, I have witnessed personal trainers new to the field improperly teaching others how to life weights in a manner that can put an individual at risk of injury. I've also witnessed others get injured as a result. This is unfortunate, but does happen. For this reason, I recommend finding out more information and getting referrals prior to hiring a personal trainer. However, if you find a qualified trainer, it can be very instrumental in helping you reach your fitness goals and keeping you on track.

Extra Nourishment when Active

When you are exercising you will want to be sure to eat plenty of nutrient rich foods to replenish your body. This will include having additional protein, healthy carbohydrates, and fat on those days that you are active. The amount will vary based on how active you are. As long as you are making healthy choices, you will do well to include the amount that feels right to you.

Exercise Prescription for Optimal Mental Health

Frequency: 3-6 times per week

Duration: 20-60 minutes

Intensity: Low to Moderate

- ✓ Find activities you enjoy
- ✓ Listen to your body
- ✓ Choose activity based on current level of fitness
- ✓ Consider having an exercise partner to keep you on track
- ✓ Consider hiring a qualified personal trainer

Chapter 17
Other Therapies

Essential Oils

Over the past year I have had the opportunity to experience the impact that essential oils can have on your health and overall well-being. Essential oils can have a profound effect on emotional health, and can help to release emotional trauma and help bring healing.

The Young Living Essential Oils Company has a Feelings Kit that can help you to heal from emotional trauma. I have found this to be a great addition to obtaining optimal mental wellness. You may want to consider the use of essential oils to lift your spirits and help heal from emotional wounds.

Light Therapy

Natural sunlight boosts the mood and helps to keep the adrenals healthy. Seasonal Affective Disorder affects many individuals, as sunlight is greatly reduced over the fall and winter months. Some individuals have had great success using light therapy. However, it is contraindicated for those with bipolar disorder. I have not used artificial light therapy, but I do get natural sunlight whenever possible. I open up all the shades as soon as I wake up in the morning, to allow the most light in and get out into the sun and fresh air as much as possible.

Music Therapy

Music has the ability to boost one's mood. The right song at the right time can put us into a great mood. I've certainly experienced this many times.

Laughter Therapy
Laughter is good like medicine (Proverbs 17:22). Find things in life to laugh at, whether it is watching comedies or reading jokes. My son and I recently had a blast in the middle of Wal-Mart, reading prank gift boxes. We were laughing so hard I was crying. What a great time! Everyone loves to laugh. Laughing boosts our natural feel good neurotransmitters.

Smiling
Just simply smiling when you are not feeling well has the power to change how you are feeling.

Fun with Friends
It is good for your spirits to be around good friends. Sharing time with friends can be very therapeutic emotionally. Be sure to choose friends who are uplifting and not Negative Nellies.

Other Therapies
Anything that helps you to relieve stress and bring peace can be therapy for you. Find things that you love to do, and continue to include them in your life on a regular basis.

My Prayer for You

I pray that God brings you the wisdom you need to find complete healing spiritually, emotionally, physically, and mentally. I pray that you find true joy and freedom from mental illness. I pray that you live a life of love, happiness, laughter, and peace. May God bless you abundantly in all that you do. May you find your purpose in life and gain much fulfillment in it. In Jesus name, Amen

There is HOPE

Never Give Up

REFERENCES

Introduction
1. Psychiatry: An Industry of Death. Citizens Commission on Human Rights. (2006). Documentary.
2. Drapeau, C.W., & Mc Intosh, J.L. (for the American Association of Suicidology). (2014). U.S.A. Suicide 2012: Official final data. Washington, DC: American Association of Suicidology, dated October 18, 2014, downloaded from http://www.suicidology.org.
3. National Alliance on Mental Illness: Suicide fact sheet. (January 2013). Arlington, VA: The National Alliance on Mental Illness. Reviewed by Ken Duckworth, M.D., & Jacob L. Freedman, M.D. Downloaded from http://www.nami.org/factsheets/suicide_factsheet.pdf.
4. American Psychiatric Association. Diagnostic and Statistical Manual on Mental Disorders, fifth edition (DSM-V). (2013). Arlington, VA: American Psychiatric Publishing.
5. Kirsch, Irving, Ph.D. (2010).*The Emperor's New Drugs: Exploding the Antidepressant Myth.* The Random House Group, Ltd. in the UK. Page 3.
6. National Institute of Mental Health: Mental Health Medications. (January 2012). Bethesda, MD: The National Institute of Mental Health. Downloaded from http://www.infocenter.nimh.nih.gov/nimh/product/mental-health-medications/nih%2012-3929 on December 10, 2014.

CHAPTER 4
Building A Healthy Mind Emotionally
1. Lyubomirsky, Sonja. (2007). *The How of Happiness*. Penguin Group, Inc., p. 15
2. Seligman, Martin, E.P. (2002). *Authentic Happiness*. New York: Free Press.

CHAPTER 5
Building A Healthy Mind Via A Healthy Nervous System
1. Genthner, C.G., Friedman, H.L., Studley, C.F. (November 7, 2005). "Improvement in Depression Following Reduction of Upper Cervical Vertebral Subluxation Using Orthospinology Technique." *Journal of Vertebral Subluxation Research.* . Pages 1-4.

2. Quigley, W.H. (June 4, 1983). "Pioneering Mental Health: Institutional Psychiatric Care in Chiropractic." *Chiropractic History* 3 (1).
3. Behrendt, M., Olsen, N. (September 20, 2004). "The Impact of Subluxations Correction on Mental Health: Reduction of Anxiety In A Female Patient Under Chiropractic Care." *Journal of Vertebral Subluxation Research*. Pages 1-10.
4. Mahanidis, T., Russell, D. (January 31, 2010). "Improvement in Quality of Life in a Patient with Depression Undergoing Chiropractic Care Using Torque Release Technique: A Case Study." *Journal of Vertebral Subluxation Research*.
5. Elster, Erin. (July 12, 2003). "Upper Cervical Chiropractic Care For A Nine-Year-Old Male With Tourette Syndrome, Attention Deficit Hyperactivity Disorder, Depression, Asthma, Insomnia, and Headaches: A Case Report." *Journal of Vertebral Subluxation Research*. Pages 1-11.
6. Wolfertz, M., Dahlberg, V. (June 20, 2012). "Upper Cervical Chiropractic Care of a Sixteen-Year-Old Male with Bipolar Disorder, Attention Deficit Hyperactivity Disorder and Vertebral Subluxation." *Journal of Upper Cervical Chiropractic Research* Issue 2. Pages 55-62.

CHAPTER 6
Building A Healthy Mind Nutritionally
1. Hoffer, A. M.D., Ph.D. (1999). *Orthomolecular Treatment for Schizophrenia: Megavitamin supplements and nutritional strategies for healing and recovery.* NTC/Contemporary Publishing Group, Inc. Lincolnwood, Illinois.
2. Ross Julia, MA. (2002). *The Mood Cure*. Penguin Group, Inc. New York, NY.

CHAPTER 7
Optimal Mental Health Nutrition Plan: Phase One, Step 1 – Nutrient Supply
1. Brogan, Kelly, M.D. (March 19, 2014) "Two Foods That May Sabotage Your Brain." *Holistic Women's Health Psychiatry* http://kellybroganmd.com/article/two-foods-may-sabotage-brain/
2. Stoll, Andrew, L., M.D. (2001). *The Omega-3 Connection*. Simon & Schuster.

3. Werbach, Melvyn R., M.D. (1999). *Nutritional Influences on Mental Illness: A sourcebook of clinical research 2nd Edition.* Third Line Press, Inc.
4. Reviewed by Derrer, David, T. (July 27, 2014). *WebMD Medical Reference.* WebMD, LLC. http://www.webmd.com/digestive-disorders/celiac-disease/celiac-disease
Viewed on 1/2/15.
5. Perlmutter, David, M.D. (2013). *Grain Brain.* Little, Brown, and Company Hachette Book Group, Inc.
6. Jackson, J., et.al. (March 2012). "Neurologic and Psychiatric Manifestations of Celiac Disease and Gluten Sensitivity." *Psychiatric Quarterly.* 83(1): 91-102.
7. Severence, E., et.al. (May 2014). "Seroreactive marker for inflammatory bowel disease and associations with antibodies to dietary proteins in bipolar disorder." *Bipolar Disorders* 16 (3): 230-240.
8. Severence, E., et.al. (May 2010). "Subunit and whole molecule specificity of the anti-bovine casein immune response in recent onset psychosis and schizophrenia." *Schizophrenia Research.* 118(1-3):240-247.
9. Campbell-McBride, Natasha, M.D. (2010). *Gut and Psychology Syndrome.* Medinform Publishing UK, p. 53-54.
10. Hoggan, Ron. (2002). *Dangerous Grains.* Pengiun Putnam, Inc, p. 148, 78.
11. Tasnime, N. Akbaraly, Ph.D. (2009). "Dietary pattern and depressive symptoms in middle age." *The British Journal of Psychiatry* 195: 408-413.

CHAPTER 8
Optimal Mental Health Nutrition Plan: Breakdown of Food Choices and Meals

1. Rubik, Beverly (Fall 2011). "How Does Pork Prepared in Various Ways Affect the Blood." *Wise Traditions in Food, Farming, and the Healing Arts.* http://www.westonaprice.org/health-topics/how-does-pork-prepared-in-various-ways-affect-the-blood/
2. Bruce, Fife. (2003). *The Healing Miracle of Coconut Oil.* Healthwise Publications.
3. Greden, J., Fontaine, P., Lubetsky, M., and Chamberlin, K. (1978). Anxiety and depression associated with caffeinism among psychiatric inpatients. *American Journal of Psychiatry*, 135 (8): 963-6.

4. Gilliland, K., and Andress, D. (1981). Ad lib caffeine consumption, symptoms of caffeinism, and academic performance. *American Journal of Psychiatry*, 138: 512-4.
5. Rapoport, J., Jensvold, M., Elkins, R., Buchsbaum, M.S., Weingartner, H., Ludlow, C., Zahn, T.P., Berg, C.I., and Neims, A.H. (1981). Behavioral and cognitive effects of caffeine in boys and adult males. *Journal of Nervous and Mental Disease*, 169: 726-732.
6. Victor, B., Lubetsky, M., and Greden. J. (1981). Somatic manifestations of caffeinism. *Journal of Clinical' Psychiatry*, 42: I85.
7. Uhde, T.W., Boulenger, J.P., Jimerson, D.C., and Post, R.M. (1984). Caffeine: Relationship to human anxiety, plasma MHPG and cortisol. *Psychopharmacology Bulletin*.20:426.
8. Roca, D.J. Schiler, G.D., and Farb, D.H. (May 1998). Chronic Caffeine or Theophyliline Exposure Reduces Gamma amminobutyric Acid/Benzodiazepine Receptor Site Interactions. *Molecular Pharmacology* 33 (5): 481-85.

CHAPTER 10
Optimal Mental Healthy Nutrition Plan: Phase One, Step 3 - Hydration

1. Armstrong LE., Ganio, MS., Casa, DJ., et. al. (2012) Mild dehydration affects mood in healthy young women. Journal of Nutrition 142 (2): 382-388.
2. Ganio, MS., Armsrong, LE., Casa, DJ., et al. (2011) Dehydration impairs cognitive performance and mood of men. British Journal of Nutrition. 106 (10): 1535-1543.
3. Lieberman, HR., Castellani, JW., Young AJ. (2009). Cognitive function and mood during acute cold stress after extended military training and recovery. Aviation Space & Environmental Medicine. 80 (7): 629-636.
4. Gopinathan, PM., Pichan, G., Sharma, VM. (1988). Role of Dehydration in Heat Stress-Induced Variations in Mental Performance. 43 (1): 15-17.
5. D'anci KE, Vibhakar A, Kanter JH, Mahoney CR, Taylor HA. (2009). Voluntary dehydration and cognitive performance in trained college athletes. Perceptual & Motor Skills. 109 (1): 251-269.

CHAPTER 11
Optimal Mental Health Nutrition Plan: Phase Two -Your Microbiome and Sleep

1. "How to Easily and Inexpensively Ferment Your Own Vegetables." (December 15, 2012). Web. *Dr. Mercola* http://articles.mercola.com/sites/articles/archive/2012/12/15/caroline-barringer-interview.aspx

2. "What is serotonin? What does serotonin do?" (September 1, 2014). Web. *Medical News Today.* http://www.medicalnewstoday.com/articles/232248.php

3. Bouchez, Colette. Reviewed by Nazario, Brunilda, MD. "Serotonin: 9 Questions and Answers." *Web MD.* Accessed 16 January 2015. http://www.webmd.com/depression/features/serotonin

4. Gershon, Michael (1998). *The Second Brain: The Scientific Basis of Gut Instinct and a Groundbreaking New Understanding of Nervous Disorders of the Stomach and Intestines.* New York, NY: Harper Collins Publishers.

5. Hadhazey, Adam. (February 12, 2010). "Think Twice: How the Gut's 'Second Brain' Influences Mood and Well-Being" *Scientific American.* http://www.scientificamerican.com/article/gut-second-brain/

6. Maes M, Kubera M, Leunis JC, Berk M. (2012). Increased IgA and IgM responses against gut commensals in chronic depression: further evidence for increased bacterial translocation or leaky gut. *Journal of Affective Disorders.* 141:55-62.

7. Maes M, Kubera M, Leunis JC. (2008). The gut-brain barrier in major depression: intestinal mucosal dysfunction with an increased translocation of LPS from gram negative enterobacteria (leaky gut) plays a role in the inflammatory pathophysiology of depression. *Neuro Endocrinology Letters.* 29:117-124

8. Alonso C, Guilarte M, Vicario M, Ramos L, Rezzi S, Marinez C, Lobo B, Martin FP, Pigrau M, Gonzalez-Castro AM, Gallart M, Malagelada JR, Azpiroz F, Kochhar S, Santos J. (2012). Acute experimental stress evokes a differential gender-determined increase in human intestinal macromolecular permeability. *Neurogastroenterology & Motility.* 24:740-746.

9. van Wijck K, Lenaerts K, Grootjans J, Wijnands DA, Poeze M, van Loon LJ, Dejong CH, Buurman WA. (2012). Physiology and pathophysiology of splanchnic hypoperfusion and intestinal injury

during exercise strategies for evaluation and prevention. *American Journal of Physiology Gastrointestinal & Liver Physiology.* 303:G155-G168.
10. Li X, Kan EM, Lu J, Cao Y, Wong RK, Keshavarzian A, Wilder-Smith CH. (2013). Combat-training increases intestinal permeability, immune activation and gastrointestinal symptoms in soldiers. *Alimentary Pharmacology & Therapeutics.* 37:799-809.
11. Messaoudi M, Lalonde R.,et. al. (2011) Assessment of psychotropic-like properties of a probiotic formulation (Lactobacillus helveticus R0052 and Bifidobacterium longum R0175) in rats and human subjects. *British* Journal of Nutrition. 105:755-764.
12. Gregoire, Carolyn. (January 4, 2015). The Surprising Link between Gut Bacteria and Anxiety. *The Huffington Post.* http://www.huffingtonpost.com/2015/01/04/gut-bacteria-mental-healt_n_6391014.html.
13. Logan AC, Katzman M. (2005). Major depressive disorder: probiotics may be an adjuvant therapy. *Medical Hypothesis.* 64:533-538.
14. Dinan TG, Stanton C, Cryan JF. (2013). Psychobiotics: a novel class of psychotropic. *Biological Psychiatry.* 74:708-709.
15. Barret E, Ross RP, O'Toole PW, Fitzgerald GF & Stanton C. (2012). Y-Aminobutyric acid production by culturable bacteria from the human intestine. Journal of Applied Microbiology. 113:411-417.
16. http://www.immunitrition.com/Organic_Cultured_Veggies.html
17. Dr. Mercola. (July 31, 2011). GAPS Nutritional Program: How a Physician Cured Her Son's Autism... Web. Dr. Mercola. http://articles.mercola.com/sites/articles/archive/2011/07/31/dr-natasha-campbell-mcbride-on-gaps-nutritional-program.aspx.

CHAPTER 12
Optimal Mental Health Nutrition Plan: Phase Three – Liver Health
1. Bennett Peter, N.D., Barrie Stephen, N.D., Faye Sara. (2001). *7-Day Detox Miracle.* Three Rivers Press. New York, NY.
2. Le Strat Yann, Le Foll Bernard, Dubertret Caroline. (2014). Major depression and suicide attempts in patients with liver disease in the United States. *Liver International.* Online ISSN 1478-3223.
3. Wilson Lawrence, M.D. (January 2014). Glutathione, Anti-Oxidants and Nutritional Balancing Science. The Center for Development. http://drlwilson.com/ARTICLES/GLUTATHIONE.htm

4. Shephard RJ, Johnson N. (Jan 2015). Effects of physical activity upon the liver. *European Journal of Applied Physiology* 115 (1):1-46.
5. Roizman Tracey, D.C. (May 22, 2011). What to Eat to Produce More Bile in the Liver. Livestrong.com. Retrieved from http://www.livestrong.com/article/448615-what-to-eat-to-produce-more-bile-in-the-liver/

CHAPTER 13
Optimal Mental Health Nutrition Plan: Phase Four, Step 1 – Hormone Health

1. Daniel Kaayla. (October 13, 2011). Sex and the Soybean. The Weston A. Price Foundation for *Wise Traditions in Food, Farming, and the Healing Arts.* http://www.westonaprice.org/blogs/kdaniel/sex-and-the-soybean-a-cautionary-tale/
2. Group Edward. (August 24, 2014). 5 Ways Soy Upsets Hormone Balance. Global Healing Center: Natural Health & Organic Living. http://www.globalhealingcenter.com/natural-health/5-ways-soy-upsets-hormone-balance
3. Siepmann T, Roofeh J, Kiefer FW, Edelson DG. (Jul-Aug 2011). Hypogonadism and erectile dysfunction associated with soy product consumption. *Nutrition.* 27(7-8):859-62.
4. Russo J, Russo IH. (Dec 2006). The role of estrogen in the initiation of breast cancer. *Journal of Steroid Biochemistry and Molecular Biology.* 102(1-5):89-96.
5. Chavarro JE, Toth TL, Sadio SM, Hauser R. (Nov 2008). Soy food and isoflavone intake in relation to semen quality parameters among men from an infertility clinic. *Human Reproduction.* 23(11):2584-90.
6. Nienhiser Jill. (August 26, 2003). Studies Showing Adverse Effects of Dietary Soy, 1939-2014. The Weston A. Price Foundation for *Wise Traditions in Food, Farming, and the Healing Arts.* http://www.westonaprice.org/health-topics/studies-showing-adverse-effects-of-dietary-soy-1939-2008/
7. Conrad S and others. (Jan 2004). Soy formula complicates management of congenital hypothyroidism. *Archives of Disease in Childhood* 89(1):37-40.
8. Wilson James. (January 15, 2015). *Cortisol and HPA Axis Function in Major Depression.* Web – Dr. James Wison's Adrenal Fatigue Blog http://blog.adrenalfatigue.org/general-health/cortisol-and-hpa-axis-function-in-major-depression/

9. Maripuu M, Wikgren M, Karling P, Adolfsson R, Norrback K-F. (2014). Relative Hypo- and Hypercortisolism Are Both Associated with Depression and Lower Quality of Life in Bipolar Disorder: A Cross-Sectional Study. *PLoS ONE* 9(6): e98682.
10. Wilson James, N.D., D.C., Ph.D. (2001). *Adrenal Fatigue: The 21st Century Stress Syndrome.* Smart Publications. Petaluma, CA.
11. Ishizuki Y, et. al. (1991). The effect on the thyroid gland of soy beans administered experimentally in healthy subjects. *Nippon Naibunpi gakkai Zasshi* 67:622-29.
12. Abdullatif HD, Ashraf AP. (Sep-Oct 2006). Reversible subclinical hypothyroidism in the presence of adrenal insufficiency. *Endocrinology Practice Journal* 12(5):572.
13. Revis NW, McCauley P, Bull R, Holdsworth G. (1986). Relationship of drinking water disinfectants to plasma cholesterol and thyroid hormone levels in experimental studies." *Proceedings of National Academy of Sciences of the United States of America.* 83:1485-89.
14. Revis NW, McCauley P, Holdsworth G. (1986). "Relationship of dietary iodide and drinking water disinfectants to thyroid function in experimental animals." *Environmental Health Perspectives.* 69:243-46.

CHAPTER 14
Optimal Mental Health Nutrition Plan: Phase Four, Step 2 - Detoxification

1. Bradbury, M., Deane, R. (1993). Permeability of the blood-brain barrier to lead. *Neurotoxicology.* 14(2-3): p. 131-6.
2. Yokel, R. (2002). Brain uptake, retention and efflux of aluminium and manganese. *Environmental Health Perspectives.* 110(5): p. 699-704.
3. Langford, N., Ferner, R. (1999). Toxicity of mercury. *Journal of Human Hypertension.* 13(10): p. 651-6.
4. Pataracchia Raymond J., B.Sc., N.D. (2008). Orthomolecular Treatment for Depression, Anxiety & Behavior Disorders. International Guide to the World of Alternative Mental Health. http://www.alternativementalhealth.com/articles/orthomolecular-anxiety-depression.htm
5. Maryse Bouchard, PhD, MSc, David C. Bellinger, PhD, MSc, and Marc G. Weisskopf, PhD (2009). Blood lead levels and major depressive disorder, panic disorder, and generalized anxiety disorder in U.S. young adults. *Archives of General Psychiatry.* 66(12): 1313-1319.
6. Rhodes D, Spiro A, 3rd, Aro A, Hu H. (2003).Relationship of bone and blood lead levels to psychiatric symptoms: the normative aging

study. *Journal of Occupational & Environmental Medicine.* 45(11):1144–1151
7. Clifton JC 2nd (2007). "Mercury exposure and public health". *Pediatric Clinics of North America.* 54 (2): 237–69,
8. Brinkel J, M.D., Khan MH, Kraemer A. (May 2009). A Systemic Review of Arsenic Exposure and its Social and Mental Health Effects with Special Reference to Bangladesh. *International Journal of Environmental Research and Public Health.* 6(5): 1609-1619.
9. Daniel Kaayla, PhD., Knight Galen, PhD. (April 2, 2009). Mad As a Hatter. The Weston A. Price Foundation for *Wise Traditions in Food, Farming, and the Healing Arts.* http://www.westonaprice.org/health-topics/mad-as-a-hatter/

CHAPTER 15
Optimal Mental Health Nutrition Plan: Phase Five – Specific Nutrients

1. Ramsey D., M.D., Muskin P., Ph.D. (January 2013). Vitamin deficiencies and mental health: How are they linked? *Current Psychiatry.* 12(1).
2. Williams Roger, Kalita Dwight. (1977). *A Physicians Handbook on Orthomolecular Medicine.* Pergamon Press Inc. Elmsford, NY. p. 184.
3. Top 10 Foods Highest in Vitamin B1 (Thiamin) Healthaliciousness.com Retrieved on 1/17/15 from http://www.healthaliciousness.com/articles/thiamin-b1-foods.php
4. Hoffer, A. M.D., Ph.D. (1999). *Orthomolecular Treatment for Schizophrenia: Megavitamin supplements and nutritional strategies for healing and recovery.* NTC/Contemporary Publishing Group, Inc. Lincolnwood, Illinois.
5. Pfeiffer Carl, PhD, MD. (1987). *Nutrition and Mental Illness: An Orthomolecular Approach to Balancing Body Chemistry.* Healing Arts Press. Rochester, Vermont. p. 21-25.
6. Top 10 Foods Highest in Vitamin B3 (Niacin) Healthaliciousness.com Retrieved on 1/17/15 from http://www.healthaliciousness.com/articles/foods-high-in-niacin-vitamin-B3.php
7. Linus Pauling Institute. Micronutrient Information Center. Retrieved on February 8, 2015 from http://lpi.oregonstate.edu/infocenter/vitamins/vitaminB6/
8. Top 10 Foods Highest in Vitamin B6. Healthaliciousness.com. Retrieved on 1/17/15 from

http://www.healthaliciousness.com/articles/foods-high-in-vitamin-B6.php
9. The Merck Manual. Folate. (Reviewed on October 2014 by Larry E. Johnson, M.D., Ph.D.) Retrieved on 1/17/15 from http://www.merckmanuals.com/professional/nutritional_disorders/vitamin_deficiency_dependency_and_toxicity/folate.html?qt=folate%20deficiency&alt=sh
10. Top 10 Foods Highest in Vitamin B9 (Folate). Healthaliciousness.com Retrieved on 1/17/15 from http://www.healthaliciousness.com/articles/foods-high-in-folate-vitamin-B9.php
11. The Merck Manual. Vitamin B12. (Reviewed on October 2014 by Larry E. Johnson, M.D., Ph.D.) Retrieved on 1/17/15 from http://www.merckmanuals.com/professional/nutritional_disorders/vitamin_deficiency_dependency_and_toxicity/vitamin_b12.html?qt=B12%20Deficiency&alt=sh
12. Top 10 Foods Highest in Vitamin B12. Healthaliciousness.com. Retrieved on 1/17/15 from http://www.healthaliciousness.com/articles/foods-high-in-vitamin-B12.php
13. Top 10 Foods Highest in Vitamin C. Healthaliciousness.com. Retrieved on 1/17/15 from http://www.healthaliciousness.com/articles/vitamin-C.php
14. The Merck Manual. Vitamin C. (Reviewed on October 2014 by Larry E. Johnson, M.D., Ph.D.) Retrieved on 1/17/15 from http://www.merckmanuals.com/professional/nutritional_disorders/vitamin_deficiency_dependency_and_toxicity/vitamin_c.html?qt=vitamin%20c%20deficiency&alt=sh
15. Top 10 Foods Highest in Magnesium. Healthaliciousness.com. Retrieved on 1/17/15 from http://www.healthaliciousness.com/articles/foods-high-in-magnesium.php
16. Greenblatt James M.D. (November 14, 2011). Psychological Consequences of Vitamin D Deficiency. *Psychology Today*. http://www.psychologytoday.com/blog/the-breakthrough-depression-solution/201111/psychological-consequences-vitamin-d-deficiency
17. The Merck Manual. Vitamin D. (Reviewed on October 2014 by Larry E. Johnson, M.D., Ph.D.) Retrieved on 1/17/15 from http://www.merckmanuals.com/professional/nutritional_disorders/vita

min_deficiency_dependency_and_toxicity/vitamin_d.html?qt=vitamin%20d%20deficiency&alt=sh
18. Top 10 Foods Highest in Vitamin D. Healthaliciousness.com. Retrieved on 1/17/15 from http://www.healthaliciousness.com/articles/high-vitamin-D-foods.php
19. Werbach, Melvyn R., M.D. (1999). *Nutritional Influences on Mental Illness: A sourcebook of clinical research 2nd Edition.* Third Line Press, Inc.
20. Stoll, Andrew, L., M.D. (2001). *The Omega-3 Connection.* Simon & Schuster.
21. Ross Julia, MA. (2002). *The Mood Cure.* Penguin Group, Inc. New York, NY.
22. Miller AL. (Sep 2008). The methylation, neurotransmitter, and antioxidant connections between folate and depression. Alternative Medicine Review. 13(3):216-26.
23. Pauling Linus. (1967). Orthomolecular Psychiatry. Center for the Study of Democratic Institutions, Santa Barbara, California. http://profiles.nlm.nih.gov/ps/access/MMBBJQ.pdf
24. Pauling Linus, Kamb Barclay. (2001). *Linus Pauling: Selected Scientific Papers, Volume II.* World Scientific Publishing Co. River Edge, NJ. p. 1364.

CHAPTER 16
Building A Healthy Mind Through Fitness
1. Li X, Kan EM, Lu J, Cao Y, Wong RK, Keshavarzian A, Wilder-Smith CH. (2013). Combat-training increases intestinal permeability, immune activation and gastrointestinal symptoms in soldiers. *Alimentary Pharmacology & Therapeutics.* 37:799-809.
2. University of Toronto Media Room. (October 25, 2013). Moderate exercise not only treats but prevents depression. http://media.utoronto.ca/media-releases/moderate-exercise-not-only-treats-but-prevents-depression/
3. Mammen G., Faulkner G. (2013). Physical Activity and the Prevention of Depression: A Systematic Review of Prospective Studies. *American Journal of Preventative Medicine.* 45(5): 649-657.
4. Exercise and Depression (2013). Harvard Health Publications Harvard Medical School. http://www.health.harvard.edu/newsweek/Exercise-and-Depression-report-excerpt.htm/

QUICK REFERENCE SHOPPING LIST
Healthy Protein Sources
- ✓ Grass-Fed Organic Beef
- ✓ Pastured or Free-Range Organic Eggs/Chicken
- ✓ Bison/Buffalo
- ✓ Venison/Deer
- ✓ Lamb
- ✓ Wild Meats
- ✓ Free-Range Organic Turkey
- ✓ Organic Nitrate-Free Ham, Pork, & Bacon
- ✓ Wild-Caught Fish/Seafood

Healthy Fat Sources
- ✓ Organic Virgin Coconut Oil
- ✓ Extra-Virgin Organic Olive Oil
- ✓ Organic Butter
- ✓ Organic Olives
- ✓ Avocados

Vegetables: All are permitted. Choose organic, local, in-season or organic frozen. Corn is a grain and is not permitted.

Fruits: All are permitted. Choose organic, local, in-season or organic frozen.

Beans: All beans are permitted. Choose dry beans and soak instead of canned.

Drinks:

- ✓ Coconut Water
- ✓ Coconut Milk
- ✓ Organic Coffee (in moderation)

Other Allowed Items

- ✓ Raw Honey
- ✓ Pure Maple Syrup
- ✓ Black Molasses
- ✓ Balsamic, Apple-Cider, or Coconut Vinegar
- ✓ Coconut Aminos
- ✓ Coconut Flour
- ✓ Gluten-Free Spices/Seasonings
- ✓ Sea Salt
- ✓ Gluten-Free Vanilla Extract
- ✓ Raw Cacao or Cocoa Powder
- ✓ Herbs & Sprouts
- ✓ Brown Rice Bread Crumbs

About the Author

Nancy Rose is a Certified Nutritional Therapy Practitioner, Certified Strength & Conditioning Specialist, Certified Healing Foods Specialist™, and a Certified GAPS™ (Gut & Psychology Syndrome) Practitioner. She has been in the fitness and nutrition field for 20 years, and has spent her life studying nutrition in order to heal herself from mental illness. Nancy is the owner & president of Get At The Roots Weight Loss, LLC and creator of the Get At The Roots Weight Loss Program with 125+ instructors in the U.S. & Canada. The Get At The Roots Program is a unique weight loss program designed to determine and correct the 10 root underlying causes of weight gain for long-term weight loss success. Instructors can be found by visiting **www.GetAtTheRootsWeightLoss.com.** Nancy is the mother of an amazing teenager, Jonathan JT Rose, who has been her inspiration to obtain health since the moment she found out she was pregnant. She currently resides in New England with her son and husband, Jimmy. Her hopes are to help as many people as possible find the freedom she has, by sharing her story. To contact Nancy regarding speaking please visit **www.GetAtTheRoots.com.**

Made in the USA
Middletown, DE
12 March 2015